LUPUS UNDERGROUND

A PATIENT'S CASE FOR A
LONG-IGNORED
DRUG-FREE
NON-PATENTABLE
COUNTER-INTUITIVE THERAPY
THAT ACTUALLY WORKS

———

A REFERENCE FOR
LUPUS UVA1 PHOTOTHERAPY RESEARCH

WRITTEN AND COMPILED BY
ANTHONY DEBARTOLO

HYDE PARK MEDIA

Printed simultaneously in the United States of America
and the United Kingdom

First Edition: November 2004

Manufacturing:
Lightning Source, LaVergne, TN • Lightning Source, Milton Keynes, UK

Book Design:
www.danielgraphics.com

ISBN 0-9763428-0-4

Published by:
HYDE PARK MEDIA
Evanston, Illinois
www.hydeparkmedia.com

To every individual ever stricken with lupus.
To every physician who has provided compassionate care.
To every family member who, too, has suffered.
And to the comforting light at the end of the tunnel.

CONTENTS

THE BASICS

If the demonstrated potential of UVA1 light to improve the lives of lupus suffer-ers were more publicly known, if research concerning both benefits and risks were accurately presented, if critics were fair, if our pharmaceutical industry didn't hold excessive power over medical research and practice, if patients were motivat-ed to take more responsibility for their own well-being, Lupus Underground would not have needed to be written — if UVA1 light didn't alleviate fatigue, it wouldn't have been.

A few weeks after the 9/11 terrorist attacks my body underwent an internal siege of its own. Lupus hit hard. My immune system went berserk. I became, in effect, allergic to myself.

After surviving the initial flare, much of the next two and a half years was spent researching a constant series of vexing new symptoms, ever on the lookout for safe and effective treatments.

In December of 2003, I boarded a New Orleans-bound sleeping car to check one out: The U.S. Food and Drug Administration (FDA)-approved clinical trial of Dr. Hugh McGrath Jr., a Professor of Rheumatology in the Department of Medicine at Louisiana State University. His treatment method, unlike all others, did not involve high-ly toxic drugs. McGrath used light — ultraviolet light.

McGrath, 68, began experimenting with ultraviolet (UV) wavelengths and lupus cells in the late 1970s, moved on to mice in the 1980s, then humans in the 1990s. While shorter UV wavelengths activated the disease, he observed that the longest band of UV wavelengths, called UVA1, mitigated the disease. The majority of lupus patients he eventually treated showed remarkable improvement. In 2001 a research team in The Netherlands published a study which claimed even better results using UVA1 than McGrath in lowering disease activity. [See Appendix B for key lupus/UVA1 research studies.]

During a quick tour of his New Orleans lab, McGrath demonstrated his UVA1 light appliance — basically, a specially outfitted commercial sun

1

tanning bed. He turned it on and I cast my swollen, achy hands under its soft light for no more than 20 seconds. Surprisingly, it felt soothing. Not a lot. But enough to notice and convince me I needed to try it.

McGrath, however, refused my entry into his tightly controlled clinical trial. It was limited to local patients, he said. Once back home, with the encouragement of my own physician, and after spending nearly six more weeks researching and exactly $4,920.48, I built my own UVA1 light appliance.

Although not pretty, given all the heat-resistant duct tape used to attach the acrylic filter, it works. And works well. My 8-bulb, 120-volt residential sun canopy matches the therapeutically effective radiation levels of the 24-lamp, 220-volt commercial sun bed in McGrath's lab.

The primary components of both devices — the lamps and filter — are the same. More than 20 years ago, they were originally developed for the sun tanning industry in Europe. So in February of 2004, I began work on my own tan.

McGrath's New Orleans patients typically received 20 minute exposures per side, two or three days per week. My own doctor suggested cutting that down to 10. I cut it to five. Despite the fact UVA1 radiation is as close to visual light, wavelength-wise, as you can get and still be called ultraviolet, it's still radiation.

The caution was rewarded. After a total of only 10 minutes I ended up slightly sunburned. McGrath's research standard of 40 minutes total would have fried me. However, five minutes per side was also all it took to provide near immediate relief of my fatigue. The energy lupus hijacked more than two years ago was back. Forget the sunburn.

Overall, McGrath's patients (about 54 total, he said, as of the Summer of 2004) also often reported fatigue as the first symptom to go, but never immediately, usually after a week or two of treatments. Reduced joint pain, inflammation, fever, morning stiffness, improved cognitive function, and decreased photosensitivity are also commonly cited.

In addition to fatigue relief, I've found UVA1 effective in reducing joint pain, inflammation and morning stiffness. After the initial flare fevers weren't an ongoing problem, so I can't attest to its effectiveness in that regard. But as for cognitive function, when I sat up after the first exposure and looked about the room, I experienced a new found sense of clarity. Not visual, but mental. And again, not a dramatic change, but enough to notice. It was as if a slight breeze had come along and swept away a cobweb from my brain that I didn't even know was there. This past summer, I've also noticed a reduction in my photosensitivity, enough to relax my dress code a bit.

At the start of my first summer trying to live with lupus, while I knew I had a need to cover up, my body didn't quite understand exactly how much. Thinking long pants and a long-sleeved shirt would suffice, I went for a short walk along Evanston's glimmering lakefront one bright June day and ended up hobbling back home after my very own personal solar flare. In 15 minutes both knees gave out and I was crippled with pain.

The rest of my summer days were spent close to home. When I did venture out I donned a broad brimmed white hat, large sunglasses, and chemically treated cotton or tightly woven polyester clothing from New Zealand designed to block UV. For complete protection, a liberal amount of sun block was applied to what was left exposed. I even buttoned the shirt's collar. On 95 degree days, I looked like a homeless pimp.

Being a research scientist and not an entrepreneur, McGrath finally got around to applying for a patent on his innovation after it was too late. Patentability is lost if more than one year before the patent application filing date, the invention was described in a printed publication. It was a few years after McGrath first published his findings in a scientific journal that he decided to apply. Consequently, the use of UVA1 light as a therapy for lupus is now in the public domain.

That, plus the fact the UVA1 light equipment employed uses off-the-shelf technology, has kept the medical device industry from beating a path to McGrath's laboratory door. If he had their support, McGrath would not now be bogged down on the road to FDA approval — stuck in Phase II multicenter clinical trials with only one research center, his own. Unless more open, this proven effective treatment with no known toxic effects, stays there.

Historically this is not a radical treatment. It should not be approached with undue caution. Hippocrates, the "Father of Medicine," used the sun as a curative agent in ancient Greece. And even he likely wasn't the first.

More recently, in 1903 Dr. Niels Ryberg Finsen received one of the first Nobel Prizes in medicine for his use of UV light in the treatment of a disease called lupus vulgaris, or tuberculosis of the skin. His work gave birth to the medical specialty of phototherapy. [See Appendix A.]

Researchers like McGrath then are not so much blazing new trails as rediscovering fertile ground overgrown with weeds. Fertilized, intentionally or not, by the pharmaceutical industry. That is not to say I am unaware of the significant lifesaving contributions to our collective health this industry has made during the past 100 years. But it is to say the industry's financial and political clout so permeates our western culture, any treatment not shaped like a pill is, well, hard to swallow.

While I am not a patient of McGrath's, he has given generously of his time to help me understand his work. My sincere thanks for the patience he has shown by never tiring of my persistent questions, or being put off by my more challenging ones. He's a Georgetown University-trained M.D., an extremely gifted and dedicated researcher, and knows as much about lupus, if not more, than any other specialist out there.

I am, however, a reporter. Not a partisan zealot. I've never taken McGrath's word as final.

There's an old motto of the famed, but now defunct Chicago News Bureau that nicely conveys my research approach — "If your mother says she loves you, check it out."

To that end I turned to Frederick Urbach, M.D., Emeritus Professor of Dermatology at Temple University, a pioneer and renowned expert in the photobiological effects of UV. He happily agreed to answer a long series of questions via e-mail. Our Q&A exchange was going to be the basis of a complete chapter for this book. "It'll give me something to do," he said. "I'm retired and don't like it very much."

My very first question was "What am I doing to my body? Am I giving myself skin cancer or what?" Urbach, who knew both McGrath and the UVA1 lupus research, said in sum, "No." Based upon the known photobiological effects of UVA1 light, and the relatively low dose of radiation employed, "there is no real risk to humans from (UVA1) therapy" for lupus, he said.

As for the treatment itself, "I have no question that it works," said Urbach. Yet the notion of clinical improvement after UVA1 is both provocative and contradictory to the maxim that UV harms lupus patients, so "When (McGrath) first started treating patients, I almost fell off my chair," he declared.

"Any idea how or why it works?" I asked. "It alters the immune status. Has an effect on antibody cells. That's as close as I can come to explaining its effectiveness," he said. "The mechanism of the effect no one has investigated 'cause it's very expensive."

Given his extensive knowledge I couldn't believe "has an effect" was all that he could say. I got the impression Urbach was holding something back. So I repeatedly pushed the point, and the obviously frustrated Urbach eventually complied: "IT KILLS IMMUNE CELLS," he bellowed. "And that's good?" I asked. "For lupus patients," he said. "But you should talk to McGrath about this." You'll find McGrath's thoughts on how UVA1 might help normalize immune responses in Chapter 4.

Urbach provided other much needed scientific clarity during our several telephone conversations and initial e-mails. But before he could complete the entire Q&A assignment, the good doctor passed away on July 8, 2004. He was 82 years young and couldn't fail to engage you, even over the phone, with his gregarious personality.

His publications were numerous, as were the awards for his research work, including the prestigious Finsen Medal of the Association Internationale de Photobiologie, and the Lifetime Achievement Award of the American Society for Photobiology.

Born in Vienna, Austria, he sounded like a scientist born in Vienna should — straight from central casting. I like to think of him as the 'Sigmund Freud of UV light,' having spent a lifetime teasing out the secrets of our sun's rays. My lessons were cut woefully short.

I also need to acknowledge and thank Chris O. Costas, M.D., referred to often in this book as "my doctor." On staff at St. Francis Hospital in Evanston, Illinois, and board certified in pediatrics, internal medicine and infectious diseases, he's not a lupus expert. But he is among the finest physicians I've met in my life, and got into the business, I think, simply to help people. He has taken wonderful care of me for more than 15 years, and was the doctor who initially hit upon the diagnosis of lupus after others were stumped. For his creative thinking, compassionate care and encouragement, I am indeed indebted.

As important as the gratitude I need to convey is this warning: Regular sun tanning beds, booths and canopies — the ones you'll find at tanning parlors across the country, or that can be purchased today for residential use — are dangerous for lupus patients. The rays emitted by these devices, even if advertised as "UVA," can trigger symptoms and make the disease much worse.

Lastly, this is not a book about lupus per se. It's a book about a long-ignored, drug-free, non-patentable, counter-intuitive therapy that I know works for me, and has reportedly helped others. While some disease basics get covered, my assumption has been that you or someone you know has lupus, and as a self-motivated individual have already done your homework. If you've recently been diagnosed, this isn't the first book you should read. In that regard, the best I've come across is *The Lupus Book: A Guide for Patients and Their Families*, by Daniel J. Wallace, Oxford University Press.

CHAPTER 1

A SLICE OF THE SUN

"The trouble with UV is that most people don't know what they're talking about."

— FREDRICK URBACH, M.D.

To understand UVA1 we need first to understand something about our sun — which is basically a ball of mainly hydrogen and helium gas. A huge ball. With a diameter of 864,000 miles, if it were hollow, more than a million Earths could fit inside.

The heat and pressure are equally immense. While the surface temperature is 6,000° C (11,000° F), temperatures at the sun's core are thought to hit 15,000,000° C (27,000,000° F). This interior heat, along with pressure of 7 trillion pounds per square inch, cause the nuclei of the hydrogen atoms to fuse, producing helium atoms in a process called fusion. This internally produced energy takes about a million years to work its way to the sun's surface before getting released into space at the speed of light in the form of electromagnetic radiation.

A standard unit of measurement for electromagnetic radiation is the size or magnitude of its wavelength — which is the distance between two successive wave crests [Figure 1]. The measurement of this distance, from long to short, varies greatly — from kilometers (km) to meters (m) to nanometers (nm). One meter equals one billion nanometers, and one nanometer is about the length of ten atoms in a row.

The spectrum of electromagnetic waves [Figure 2] ranges from very long radio wavelengths the size of buildings — followed by microwaves, infrared, visual light, ultraviolet and x-rays — to very short gamma-rays whose wavelengths are smaller than the size of an atom's nucleus. The shorter the wavelength, the greater the energy.

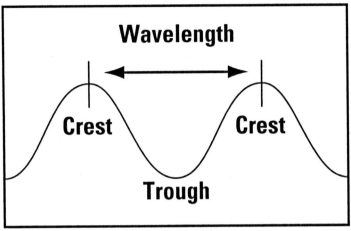

Figure 1 — wavelength

The visible light waves, which range from 400 nm to 700 nm, are the only electromagnetic waves we can see. And we see these waves as the colors of the rainbow, with each color having a different wavelength. Red has the longest and violet the shortest. When all the waves are seen together, they make white light.

Of the solar radiation that hits the top of our atmosphere, approximately 9 percent is UV, 41 percent is visual and 50 percent infrared, which is light so red we can't see it but can sense it as heat. All but 45 percent of solar radiation gets reflected back into space or is absorbed by our atmosphere.

The type of radiation we're concerned with — UV — resides between the visible light region of the electromagnetic spectrum and x-rays. UV wavelengths run from approximately 100 nm to 400 nm. And although these waves are invisible to the human eye, some insects, such as bumblebees, can see them.

UV in turn can be subdivided into three regions, based upon the known biological effects each radiation band produces. According to Urbach, these are the most often used standards:

UVA — between 400 nm and 320 nm
UVB — between 320 nm and 280 nm
UVC — between 280 nm and 100 nm

[See Figure 3]

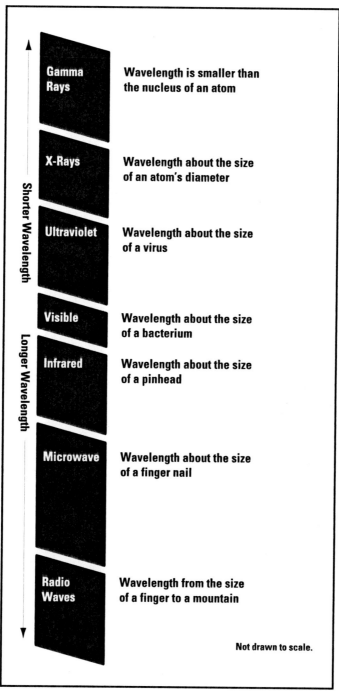

Figure 2 — an approximation of the electromagnetic spectrum

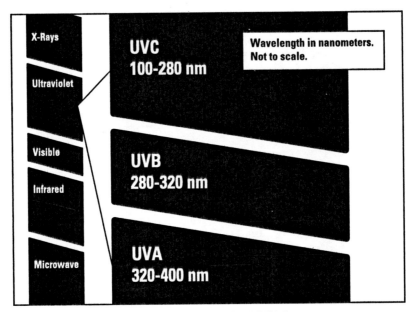

Figure 3 — UVA/UVB/UVC

Much of the sun's UVB radiation, largely responsible for our summer sunburns, gets absorbed in the ozone and oxygen molecules in our upper atmosphere, called the stratosphere. UVC, which has a wavelength energy range just below that of x-rays, gets absorbed completely in the stratosphere. If it didn't, you'd think twice about that Fourth of July picnic. Even small doses of UVC burn skin rapidly.

UVA radiation, on the other hand, is only slightly affected by stratospheric ozone levels and most of what is emitted by the sun reaches the earth's surface. According to data provided by Urbach, of the solar radiation that finally makes it to the surface around noon during the summer in North America, only about 6.3 percent is UV. Of this, 94 percent is UVA and 6 percent is UVB. Also most fortunate for our skin.

Researchers in the 1920s first discovered it took 500 to 1,000 times more energy to produce a sunburn with UVA radiation (366 nm), than it did with UVB (297 nm). Sixty years later, researchers began to realize the shorter wavelengths of the UVA range produced biological effects more like UVB than UVA's longer wavelengths. Based upon these findings, said Urbach, in 1985 noted Harvard Medical School researcher T.B. Fitzpatrick recommended subdividing the UVA range into two parts [Figure 4]:

UVA1 — between 400 nm and 340 nm
UVA2 — between 340 nm and 320 nm

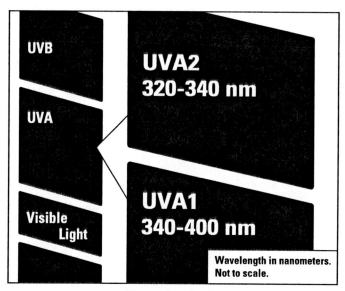

UVB

UVA

UVA2
320-340 nm

Visible
Light

UVA1
340-400 nm

Wavelength in nanometers.
Not to scale.

Figure 4 — UVA1

While the amount of UVA and UVB hitting the Earth's surface varies by latitude, altitude, time of year (and day), as well as weather conditions and pollution levels, the vast majority of the solar radiation that ends up hitting your skin on a percentage basis, is UVA1. In one measurement taken on June 21, 2003 in Tucson, AZ, UVA1 accounted for 80.7 percent, while UVA2 accounted for 15.4 percent. UVB made up 3.9 percent.

But percentages alone don't tell us much. To best comprehend the amount of radiation a person receives from the sun, a photomedical treatment or a sun tanning booth, we need a different measure. And there are two. Radiation received can be expressed in either physical energy units, or biological units.

Evaluating UV in terms of the biological effect which it produces, rather than the energy involved, is expressed as MED units, or Minimal Erythemal Dose. That's defined as the effective UV dose that causes a perceptible reddening of previously unexposed skin. You know, sunburn.

For my purpose, which was to compare the amount of UVA1 light a person would be exposed to on a typical summer day with the amount received during a typical lupus treatment, the measurement of energy is the most appropriate. These energy units are called Joules per square meter/centimeter, or Watts per square meter/centimeter, and are expressed in the following formula: Energy (Joule) = Power (watt) x Exposure Time (in seconds).

I asked Urbach to do the math. He explained that the UVA (thus UVA1) intensity at noon during the summer in our northern U.S. latitude is 5 milliwatts per centimeter squared, or 5 mWatts/cm². To convert first to millijoules one has to multiply the watts by the time in seconds. Thus, an hour's dose of UVA1 from the sun around noon is: 3600 x 5 = 18000 mJ/cm², which equal 18 Joules/cm². The lupus treatment dose is typically 6 Joules/cm², or about 1/3rd of the UVA1 radiation you'd get during the noon hour in Chicago around late June. The lupus dose, added Urbach, is "also 20 percent of a Minimal Erythemal Dose for UVA, which is 30 J/cm²."

Wanting a more apples-to-apples comparison, I did the math to see how much UVA1 radiation I'd be getting during a 9 minute treatment compared to 9 minutes in the sun. Nine minutes, or 540 seconds, works out to 2.7 Joules/cm². With my home sun baths at about 6 Joules/cm², that meant receiving 2.2 times as much UVA1 under the canopy as from the summer sun.

(Technical Note: When I write about my 8-lamp sun canopy generating 6 Joules, that's an approximation due to an inherent energy variation of the bulbs. The 6-foot long TL/10R lamps McGrath and I use have sweet spots. According to my UVA milliwatt meter readings, which I use to regulate exposures, the tube's highest energy output is concentrated in the center and falls off toward the ends. A treatment might deliver 5.97 Joules at the chest, 4.72 at calf, and 5.0 at the head.)

Receiving 2.2 times as much UVA1 during an artificial sun bath as I would outdoors struck me as relatively safe, given the fact tanning salon patrons often expose themselves to radiation levels 10 times what they'd get naturally. Still, the arguably risky behavior of "tanorexics" doesn't offer much confidence as a baseline.

In terms of comparative safety, a more reassuring example than tanners are the patients being treated for severe atopic dermatitis, a chronically relapsing skin disorder thought to involve the immune system. UVA1 phototherapy has proven to be remarkably effective for this skin disease in recent years. And as Urbach pointed out, they often use very high radiation levels of 130 Joules/cm². "The very large dose of UVA1 used for atopic dermatitis is arrived at after many treatments, so that skin has time to adjust," he explained. "I know of no published data showing (130 Joules/cm²) to be dangerous."

There is another light therapy called PUVA, Urbach added, that does have well-documented dangers and that shouldn't be confused or meaningfully compared with UVA1. That's because PUVA is not strictly a phototherapy, it's a photochemotherapy. Patients are first given psoralens, drug compounds found in many plants which make the skin temporarily sensitive to UVA before they're exposed. PUVA has been shown to increase the risk for skin cancer, including melanoma, a highly malignant and sometimes fatal form. Those who receive long-term treatments are carefully monitored throughout their lives..

In addition to the sun providing our human race with many of its first gods — Ra among the Egyptians, Helios for the Greeks, Mithras for the Persians, Apollo for the Romans, Huitzilopochtli for the Inca — its power was likely noted by the first of our kind to venture into the light from the shade of a tree or the shadow of a cave and return with a nice sunburn.

Its power has always been with us, and much has been written about both the beneficial and harmful aspects of UV. Contributing to that endless debate is not the intention here. I'll leave that to others like Michael Holick, M.D., whose new book, *The UV Advantage* (iBooks, 2004), has created an uproar, in part because some of his research was reportedly funded by the tanning industry.

Holick, a leading Vitamin D researcher, argues that regular and moderate exposure to sunlight (UVB in particular) can be good because it helps the body manufacturer the "sunshine vitamin." A deficit of this nutrient has been linked to not only osteoporosis, but breast, colon, and prostate cancer, multiple sclerosis, arthritis and hypertension.

An apparent underpinning of Holick's theory, and most others that make a case for the beneficial aspects of UV, is the concept of "hormesis," derived from the Greek word "hormaein" which means "to excite." It describes dose-response relationships in biological systems as displaying a positive effect at low doses, and a negative effect at high doses. Meaning, a little can still be good when a lot is bad.

Professor Edward Calabrese, a toxicologist at the University of Massachusetts, came up with the hormesis concept after reviewing thousands of studies that were focused on finding the negative effects of various toxins. He saw a pattern in those studies the original researchers either missed or ignored — that a little exposure to toxins, including arsenic, mercury and radiation — can have beneficial effects on both people and plants.

While we can't ignore the known or theoretical dangers of any UV radiation, Calabrese's work makes possible the theory that some might actually help. McGrath's work shows that also includes lupus patients. As initially counter-intuitive as that might seem.

CHAPTER 2

A PERSONAL JOURNEY

Lupus, as you likely know, is a chronic, inflammatory, autoimmune disorder that ranges in severity from life-threatening to life-diminishing. As you might also know, even when a case is considered minor, it's a major pain.

While a healthy immune system produces proteins called antibodies that help fight and destroy viruses, bacteria, and any other foreign substances that dare to invade, with lupus, the immune system produces antibodies against the body's own perfectly healthy cells and tissues.

These autoantibodies, as they're called, can lead to chronic inflammation of and damage to joints, skin, kidneys, heart, lungs, blood vessels, the central nervous system and brain. It can also involve connective tissue in many parts of the body as well as blood cells. The manifest symptoms often differ from patient to patient and may come and go over time. New symptoms may also continue to appear many years after the initial diagnosis.

While symptoms can differ widely, some of the more common include unexplained spikes in fever, arthritis, skin rashes, mouth and nasal sores, extreme sensitivity to sunlight, and a chronic fatigue no amount of sleep can abate.

The text books will tell you there are three types of lupus:

Discoid, or Cutaneous — Primarily limited to the body's largest organ, the skin.

Systemic Lupus Erythematosus (SLE or LE) — Considered the most common and the deadliest, it can involve all of the systems and organs mentioned above.

Drug-induced — Thought to be caused by certain prescription medications taken for other troubles, its symptoms can mirror those associated with SLE. The most common offending drugs are procainamide, used to treat heart arrhythmias, hydralazine for high blood pressure, and dilantin used to control seizures. Also on the "drug watch list" are ibuprofen and penicillin. Recently added are the powerful cholesterol-reducing drugs called statins.

Although text books neatly divide lupus into these three tidy packages, bodies don't read. A person can move back and forth between lupus types, and can develop a wide variety of related immune disorders. Irritable bowel syndrome and Crohn's disease, for example, can affect the gastrointestinal tract. Fibromyalgia can cause muscle pain. Sjögren's Syndrome can affect moisture producing glands, while Raynaud's Syndrome can impair blood vessels.

Little wonder an estimated 40 percent of lupus patients will stop working within the first year of their diagnosis. And women are the hardest hit. According to The Lupus Foundation of America, Inc., of the estimated 1.5 million people in the U.S. who suffer from this general autoimmune disorder, approximately 90 percent are female. Of those, many are women of color — either African-American, Hispanic, Asian or American Indian.

There is no cure in sight, primarily because no one knows what causes it or how lupus actually works. Autoimmune disorders in general are baffling.

The drug treatments employed when the inflammation gets out of hand are highly toxic and can have side effects that rival the damage caused by the disease itself. As for new treatments, there hasn't been one developed in decades.

The treatments available today are for symptoms, not the disease. And the mainstay are corticosteroids, used to reduce inflammation and immune system activity. But this potent hormone can also weaken or damage bones, cause high blood pressure, artery damage, diabetes, changes in physical appearance, mood and personality, as well as cataracts and infections. Infections, by the way, in and of themselves are a leading cause of death among lupus patients.

Used in the most severe cases are a group of drugs also used to treat cancer called immune suppressants, which in effect shut down the entire immune system. Among the side effects: nausea, vomiting, hair loss, bladder problems, decreased fertility and an increased risk of cancer and infection.

The most commonly used class of drugs — antimalarials — were, as the name implies, originally used to treat parasitic infections like malaria. Plaquenil (hydroxychoroquine) seems to be the antimalarial of choice. Clinical evidence suggests it can be useful in treating several symptoms, particularly those involving the skin and joints.

A list of Plaquenil's potential negative effects, though, seems longer than the positive: abdominal cramps, anemia, blisters in mouth and eyes, blood disorders, blurred or foggy vision, convulsions, diarrhea, diminished reflexes, dizziness, excessive coloring of the skin, eye muscle paralysis, halos around lights, headache, hearing loss, heart problems, hives, involuntary eyeball movement, irritability, itching, light flashes and streaks, light intolerance, liver problems or failure, loss of hair, loss or lack of appetite, muscle paralysis, muscle weakness and wasting, nausea, nervousness, nightmares, psoriasis, ringing in the ears, skin inflammation and scaling, skin rash, vertigo, vomiting and weight loss. Known to cause damage to the retina, all patients taking Plaquenil get an eye exam every 6 months.

The known deadly side effects of prescription drugs are the fourth leading cause of death in the industrialized world, surpassed only by the number of deaths from heart attacks, cancer and strokes (Journal of the American Medical Association, April 15, 1998). This fact is no surprise either, because drug patents are primarily issued for new synthetic molecules. All synthetic molecules need to be detoxified and eliminated from the body, a system that frequently fails and results in an epidemic of severe and deadly side effects.

– Dr. Rath Health Foundation
www4.dr-rath-foundation.org

A pill, by the way, is what first introduced me to lupus. More than a decade ago a prescription for something else caused the drug-induced variety to appear. And with it, crippling arthritis, pleurisy and sudden temperature spikes of 103 degrees.

I was told at the time I had lupus, but "not really." Also according to the textbooks, once the suspected drug is stopped, unlike discoid or SLE, the drug-induced variety "usually" goes away. And mine did. After a short, but difficult to tolerate course of steroids, things returned to normal. For more than a decade, I felt fine. Until the Fall of 2001 when my immune system went berserk again, only more so. But the possibility of having lupus didn't even cross my mind.

When I first saw my doctor and heard about the battery of lab tests he wanted, he also suggested one for HIV, just to be safe, he said. Coming from a general practitioner who hadn't seen a lot of AIDS patients, I wouldn't have found that advice alarming. But my doctor, among other things, is an infectious disease expert. What did he know that he wasn't telling me?

"I don't know what you have," was his straight answer. "But the sooner we find out the better."

The pharmacy clerk at my local Walgreen's, however, seemed convinced. I went to the hospital's lab for the blood and urine tests, but opted for an at-home HIV screening kit and appeared at her counter looking very much like the sick man that I was — flushed, trembling and in a heavy sweat. The $50 test kit sat in a box on a shelf behind her. I pointed, ordered one, paid cash. She rang up the sale, threw the change and receipt into a bag, pushed it across the counter, turned on her heels and disappeared into a back room. Still, she wasn't as nervous as I was a few days later when able to call the home testing kit's 800 phone number, punch in a long code and hear the results. I went to my doctor's office to make the call. "If it's positive," I told him, "I'm going to need a few Valium." Before the call, he checked the hospital's computer for the other lab results. After studying those, he said, "Anthony, I think you might have lupus."

Having an autoimmune disease instead of an acquired immune disease I immediately took as good news. Ten years earlier this same man told me "you have lupus" and it went away. After making the call and hearing that the home test result was indeed negative, my relief was complete. But short lived. It didn't take long to realize this new disease was going to stay, even though we weren't sure what to call it.

There is no single laboratory test that is used to diagnose and evaluate lupus — meaning, no single test can either prove or rule it out. The disorder is characterized by abnormalities in many test results — blood cell abnormalities, measurements for autoimmunity via specific autoantibodies, and tests for kidney disease.

Complicating the clinical picture even further is the fact that a patient can have severe symptoms with few abnormal lab results. And vice versa. The course of the disease is both unpredictable and individualized. No two patients are exactly alike. The flip side of this 'difficult to diagnose' problem is the 'difficult to treat' one. Both issues were raised by the *Wall Street Journal* in an April 15, 2004 front page story concerning the lack of new lupus drugs.

"Lupus," the report noted, "was in a vast wasteland of drug development for a striking and little-recognized reason: It's not easy to clearly measure progress in treating patients."

I went to see one of the leading lupus specialists in Chicago to learn what specific treatment plan I should follow. I brought along a folder of recent test results, as well as tests taken a decade earlier when we knew for certain it was drug-induced.

The American College of Rheumatology has established another set of diagnostic criteria that's often used — a list of 11 symptoms. If a patient has at least four of the 11, it's then considered "likely" that individual has SLE:

- Malar rash
- Discoid rash
- Photosensitivity
- Oral ulcers
- Arthritis
- Serositis (pleuritis or pericarditis)
- Renal disorder
- Neurological disorder
- Hematologic disorder
- Immunologic disorder
- Abnormal ANA titer

However, a diagnosis of lupus can still be made if a patient has fewer than four of these symptoms. As I discovered while sitting on the examining table, you can walk in with five, including the signature butterfly face rash, and still be told you don't have lupus. "Undifferentiated autoimmune disorder," the Chicago specialist said.

My own doctor, along with the new specialist he then suggested we consult, didn't know what else to call it other than lupus. Yet giving it an official name didn't offer much comfort. Neither did my new specialist's severity assessment: On a 1 to 10 point scale, he gave it a 4. Given my harsh experience, I couldn't imagine what an 8 felt like.

Over the course of the next two years, though, I got a better idea — the disorder only grew worse. Not so much in terms of the severity of symptoms, but in their type and kind. At least one morning each week it seemed I awoke with a new problem. They ran from immediately troublesome to potentially dangerous in a seemingly never ending series. Yet the symptom that sidelined me from life was the constant fatigue. Never experienced anything even remotely like it.

Nonetheless, when I felt I could safely work out my ailing body, I did. I had been working out near daily for years, and it clearly helped when lupus hit. As my doctor once said, "If you were a couch potato, you'd still be on the couch."

I was power walking on a treadmill 3 to 5 miles, 6 or 7 days a week before lupus. During the first few weeks after, I needed to be led around the block by the hand. Today I'm back up to 3 miles, 4 or 5 days a week. Meaning, I don't push it. The disease is still active. And while I report fatigue relief, at this point, I still get tired. Although there are essential qualitative and quantitative differences. If I take an afternoon nap now it's considerably shorter and I awake refreshed. Before UVA1, napping 4 hours like a sick puppy and still waking up fatigued was not unusual.

When not napping or working out, much of my time those first two lupus years was spent looking for a way out — always on the lookout for safe, effective treatments for this disease and its many conditions. Based upon that research I've started, then dropped, a few daily supplements.

I stopped taking DHEA (dehydroepiandrosterone) about a month after starting this steroid hormone made from wild yam extracts. It's naturally produced by the adrenal glands in all mammals and is used by the body to make the powerful sex hormones testosterone and estrogen. DHEA levels are known to be low in lupus patients.

The energy boost was immediate, especially for the libidinal variety, which made up for the pimple or two that came with it. But I felt the initial pharmaceutical-quality dose of 25 mg a day was just too potent. I cut back to 10 mg, then 5 mg, and then lost all positive effects. While the initial testosterone boost was nice, the parallel rise in estrogen was problematic. Given the proven link between elevated estrogen levels and prostate cancer in men, I thought it wise to look elsewhere for relief.

Among the supplements I'm still taking that I have the most confidence in is glucosamine sulfate (750 mg twice a day) for joints, especially the knees. For general inflammation, Norwegian salmon oil (1000 mg twice a day) also seems to work, at least some. I had been taking another oil for inflammation, flaxseed, but stopped after learning some studies found a link between the alpha-linolenic acid in the oil and an increased risk of prostate cancer.

A word of warning about the wonder drug aspirin. It's among several non-steroidal anti-inflammatory drugs often used by lupus patients, but it needs to be taken in relatively high doses to affect inflammation. I was up to 9 a day. Pushed it to 12 once, but cut back immediately when my ears started ringing. Today, I usually get by on one or two. I've also recently stopped taking Plaquenil after more than two years, and left behind the slight visual problems those dog-bone-shaped tablets occasionally produced.

That's because in December of 2003 my research led me to Dr. Hugh McGrath Jr., and to what I think has been the most effective intervention of all — UVA1 light.

My use of the term "effective" is not strictly subjective. McGrath, a professor at Louisiana State University in New Orleans, has successfully completed Phase I of his FDA-approved clinical trial, which is designed to determine toxicity, a safe dosage range, and offer proof that the intervention actually works. Phase I trials are the first test in a human population, usually following lab mice, and are limited to relatively few subjects. McGrath used about 50 total.

Currently, McGrath is technically in Phase II of his clinical trial, which is supposed to be carried out at multiple research centers using a few hundred subjects to further test efficacy and obtain additional data on the treatment's safety.

For the record, there's usually a Phase III and Phase IV clinical trial as well. During Phase III the research is expanded to a few thousand subjects and is designed to gather additional evidence of efficiency, monitor side effects and compare it to other commonly used treatments. Phase IV is a post-marketing study of an FDA-approved treatment designed to determine the long-term effects on morbidity and mortality.

McGrath's frustration at being stuck in Phase II with only one research center — his own — was evident shortly after we met in New Orleans. As mentioned, he isn't much of an entrepreneur. By the time McGrath got around to apply for a patent on his innovation, it was too late. To date, his research has been supported by a patchwork of relatively small grants. Without a registered patent to interest some segment of the medical industry, expanding Phase II clinical trials becomes difficult. And believing you have a simple treatment that could benefit many patients without a way to deliver it, is for a doctor, understandably frustrating.

I recall McGrath complaining about the fact that as a licensed physician, he wasn't in a position to either give or sell his equipment to other doctors for treatment purposes, let alone directly to patients for at-home use. "But I could open up a sun tanning parlor tomorrow and do the same thing," he said.

He wasn't exaggerating. Exposing one's body to UVA1 light in a commercial sun tanning bed wouldn't be anything new. When I returned from New Orleans and started researching the best way to build my own UVA1 light appliance, I discovered that the two key components of McGrath's tanning bed — the lamps and filter — were first developed and marketed for the sun tanning industry.

The lamps are made by Philips Lighting, a division of The Netherlands-based Royal Philips Electronics. According to their website: "The #1 household light bulb maker in the world." The 6-foot long lamps we use are called the TL/10R.

They used to be called the R-UVA lamp when first introduced many years ago as part of Philips world-wide tanning lamp lineup. An old sales brochure, headlined "Faster tanning without burning," put it this way: "...perhaps most important, R-UVA lamps are lined with the newly developed 'Color 10' phosphor which emits less than 0.1% UVB radiation compared to UVA. With this new phosphor, the shorter UVA wavelengths are also reduced to less than 0.1% — reducing the degree of 'sun burning' to virtually zero." [See Figure 5 for the spectral power distribution of a TL/10R lamp.]

While the lamp is important in that it produces nearly all of its wavelengths in the desired UVA1 range, it still emits a small amount of UVB and UVA2 which must be removed due to safety concerns. Consequently, the single most important component of my UVA1 light appliance is the acrylic filter, also originally created for the sun tanning industry.

(Note: McGrath's very first study with human subjects used unfiltered TL/10R lamps and considerable improvement without toxic effects were reported as short-term findings. However, given the link between skin cancer and UVB, which the TL/10R emits along with UVB-like UVA2 waves, an unfiltered treatment method would be ill advised as a practical matter. The long-term treatment regime required by lupus patients would likely make this a toxic procedure.)

The UVA1 filter was developed in 1978 by a Ph.D. optical engineer, Dr. Maxim F. Mutzhas, for the German tanning market. Mutzhas's company also produced high-performance UV irradiation systems for research, diagnosis and therapy in dermatology and pediatrics. They also manufactured electric signs.

Mutzhas, who passed away several years ago, was a close personal friend and colleague of Urbach. Urbach told me it was he who first did a spectral analysis of Mutzhas's UVA1 filter, documenting that it functioned as advertised.

One ad pitched Mutzhas's new sun tanning system this way: "A healthy tan is an important indication of people's well-being these days. And Mutzhas UVASUN tanning systems are the ultimate instrument for this. Amazingly fast, immediately visible and unusually long-lasting…The underlying principle is always 'tanning in the shade.' UVB radiation and the short-wave UVA2 are filtered out. The light and the infrared radiation are reduced…For healthy, comfortable tanning without sun burn."

Because UVA1 wavelengths penetrate deeper into the skin than UVB (but not as much as the even longer wavelengths of visual light) and are able to oxidize melanin granules farther away from the surface of the skin, it was thought these granules would take longer to reach the skin's surface and allow a tan to be deeper, darker and longer-lasting. At least that's what Mutzhas thought. His tanning innovation never really caught on, industry sources say, because it didn't work very well.

Yet an off-shoot of Mutzhas's method is firmly entrenched today in

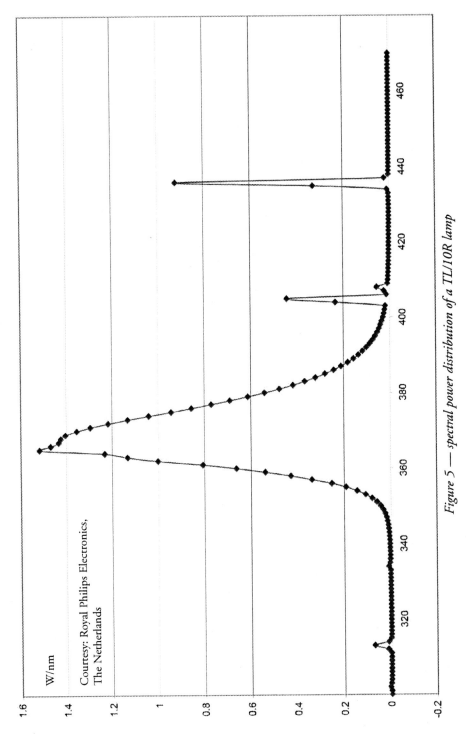

Figure 5 — spectral power distribution of a TL/10R lamp

the sun tanning industry. It's called "high-pressure" tanning because these systems utilize lamps filled with mercury vapor that can develop very high UV intensity levels. But these systems no longer deliver strictly UVA1. They now use the total UVA wavelength range and toss in some UVB. "Just enough UVB to stimulate the melanin production required and a lot of UVA to really oxidize that melanin and turn it golden brown," reads the ad copy for one high-pressure tanning bed.

Interestingly, the overall intensity of the UV emitted from several high-pressure beds I found online, was about 10 times what I'm using. The filtered TL/10R lamps I lie under are 100 watts each. Many high-pressure beds come equipped with 1,000 watt bulbs, usually 24 of them. You could roast a chicken in your lap.

The UVA1 light appliance that I ended up putting together, an 8-bulb residential sun canopy (in effect, the top half of a sun tanning bed), might be considered a "low-pressure" unit. Which may explain why I don't have much of a tan — actually a good thing because a tan is a sign of skin damage. I am, however, half a shade darker than when I started.

Lousy tan or not, hypothetically, let us suppose McGrath did open up that sun tanning parlor. He'd still be dealing with the FDA. Because the use and sale of medical devices in the treatment of disease, as well as the use and sale of sun tanning equipment in the treatment of vanity, are both regulated in the U.S. by the same federal agency, the FDA. The regulations governing medical devices, however, are more complex and expensive to satisfy than the regulations governing sun tanning equipment.

From the FDA's website: "FDA regulates radiation emitting electronic products. The purpose is to prevent unnecessary exposure to radiation due to the use of these products. There are specific requirements that apply to all radiation emitting electronic products in order to comply with the provisions of the Food, Drug and Cosmetic Act. If the product is also a medical device, the product must also comply with the medical device regulations."

Apparently, it all depends upon what you call it.

Based upon the FDA's definitions offered in "Title 21, Chapter 1, Subchapter J" of the agency's "Performance Standards for Light-Emitting Products," a UVA1 light appliance is a "Sunlamp product." Meaning, "any electronic product designed to incorporate one or more ultraviolet lamps and intended for irradiation of any part of the living human body, by ultraviolet radiation with wavelengths in air between 200 and 400 nanometers, to induce skin tanning."

At the same time, the UVA1 light appliance used by Dr. McGrath is a medical device. All of which seemed a little contradictory. Especially after discovering among the three classes of radiation emitting electronic products the FDA regulates, sun tanning beds are considered Class 1 devices, subject to the least regulatory control because they're thought to present minimal potential harm to the user.

So I called the FDA. And according to spokesperson Sharon Snider, there is no regulatory conflict. A UVA1 light appliance could exist as both a sun tanning product and as a medical device. "You mean, someone could manufacture these devices and sell them as sun tanning equipment, as long as no medical claims were made?" I asked.

"That is correct," Snider said, adding that if the same device were sold to lupus patients as a treatment, "they would be classified as a medical device." It just depends what you call it.

But calling it a "sunlamp product" doesn't mean medical safeguards can be ignored. No tanning method, other than the spray-on variety, can be considered risk-free.

There's ample evidence to suggest that in mice, at least, total UVA causes premature aging of the skin by penetrating the deepest layers and damaging the collagen — the spongy protein that gives skin its structure, firmness and elasticity. We don't know how well that might also hold true for UVA1 and humans. As Urbach put it, "We can't experiment on humans, not because it's dangerous or unethical, but because it would take too damn long — 50 years."

Before beginning the sun baths, as a baseline check I underwent a head-to-toe exam by my dermatologist. Who, after a brief debate, gave me his blessing to proceed. The issue was not that he thought UVA1 was harmful. The issue was that he didn't know what UVA1 was. Most dermatologists in daily practice don't. UVA1 just doesn't come up.

The plan was to give myself a self-exam every week, and come back in 6 months. Within two weeks of my first treatment, however, I was back in his office for a biopsy. Immediately after treatment #2 a strange multi-colored lesion appeared on my left arm, about 1/8th of an inch in diameter.

"Well," I thought, "it was sweet while it lasted."

Turned out to be a benign lichenoid keratosis, and was told not to worry. Had more to do with my age, the dermatologist said, than the UVA1. An explanation I didn't quite buy given my facts: a) the lesion was not on my arm before treatment #2, and b) it was within minutes after.

The keratosis incident was among the first things I asked Urbach about. "Your spot got dark when exposed to the light," he said. "You had it all along. You must be light skinned."

"Yes, despite the Italian surname, I am. Have some red hair and a lot of freckles, too," I replied.

"Then you have some Celt genes in you," he announced, beginning a brief European history lesson: Celtic tribes invaded Italy and established a city they called Mediolanum, which is modern day Milan. They ended up sacking Rome itself in 390 B.C. The Roman armies didn't get rid of them until 192 B.C. "Some of your ancestors must be from north of Milan," concluded Urbach. "Those genes make you burn."

The *very* first thing I asked Urbach was if there was any established link between UVA1 and cancer. His short answer was "No." Unlike UVB, UVA1 "does no damage to DNA," and skin cancer is thought to be caused by damaged DNA, he said. "I don't know of any toxic effects."

But there were two disturbing studies I found that seemingly did find a cancer link to UVA1 — one involved a specific genus of fish called *Xiphophorus*, the other, what I call bald lab mice. I e-mailed my concerns about these studies and Urbach wrote back:

"The experimental studies in mice were done with hairless (not bald) mice. However, it required very large doses and few tumors were induced...The fish story is very complicated...I do not give much credibility to it. The fish used were genetically programmed to develop melanoma." In fact, explained Urbach, visual light also induced cancer in these fish.

"We know virtually nothing about UVA and melanoma in man," he continued. "The exception are a few papers suggesting that tanning with UVA results in (melanoma). Those are questionable and this was total UVA plus some UVB. The data about UVA1 and skin cancer are again from hairless mice, and has shown a much lesser effect than that of UVB."

When I asked McGrath for his view on the UVA1/cancer/mice connection, he said simply, "You can spit on these mice and give 'em cancer."

I never asked Urbach if he agreed with that sentiment, but UVA1 he proclaimed, "is virtually non-carcinogenic. If there is any, it's almost non-existent." All things considered, "I still think that there is no real risk to humans from (UVA1) therapy for LE," he offered.

Before I spoke with Urbach, caution kept my initial sun baths to a minimum. At first, just a couple of minutes every other week. But after 3 or 4 days symptoms would always creep back, so I began a weekly schedule. The results were better, but the continuity of relief was still off. It wasn't until after speaking with Urbach that I gained the confidence to begin a schedule more in keeping with what McGrath had done in his lab — 2 or 3 times each week.

Despite Urbach's assurances, yet keeping his Celt gene theory in mind, I began to take a few more extra protective measures during the more frequent exposures. Because there was no research ever conducted on UVA's effect on a man's reproductive organs, I began double coverage there from day one. But after speaking with Urbach I started covering an arm, the back of both hands and my entire face.

While a fair complexion seems to be a potential liability, it's apparently also an advantage — the lack of melanin allows UVA1 rays to penetrate deeply, as far as the deeper layers of the dermis — that thick connective tissue immediately beneath the skin's outermost layer that contains blood and lymph vessels, sweat glands and nerve endings.

Although not specifically researched in any of McGrath's studies, his clinical observations suggest the therapy doesn't work as well for dark skinned individuals as it does for those with light complexions. It's assumed the relatively greater amount of melanin in dark skin blocks penetration. So treatment success seems to fall along racial lines.

For lupus patients as a general population that poses a significant, but not necessarily insurmountable problem. A large percentage of lupus sufferers are African-American. McGrath thinks a way to improve treatment efficiency among these patients is not through the use of photosensitizing drugs as with PUVA therapy, but by increasing the relatively low radiation level employed.

One who didn't benefit much from the original research dose was Tania, a 46-year-old African-American woman who was a subject in

McGrath's Phase I clinical trial. "I did it for 6 or 8 weeks," she said during a telephone interview from her New Orleans home. "That was back in 1989. It was a long time ago, so I don't remember exactly how long I was in the study, but I did complete it."

That was also the year Tania discovered she had lupus. "I had (joint) symptoms for about 10 years before then," she said, "but they were mild and tolerable. Besides, arthritis ran in my family so I thought it was normal. But it kicked in so bad I had to pay attention."

The pain grew so great Tania ended up in an emergency room. "The doctor there suggested I see McGrath, because it looked like lupus to him. I've been (McGrath's) patient ever since."

During the treatments, while lying in the sun bed, "I felt good in there," said Tania. "It was relaxing. It almost put me to sleep."

"When I left I was walking better. I had no pain. But a few hours later my symptoms came back," she said. "The joint pain diminished a lot, but it only lasted a few hours."

There was, however, another problem. "I got a rash from the UVA1. Sort of like prickly heat that turned into dry skin," she added.

(Note: There is a condition caused by sunlight that's particularly common in lupus patients called polymorphic light eruption, or PLE. It's also know as "prickly heat." This could very well be what happened to Tania, but it occurred so long ago, neither she nor McGrath could remember the actual diagnosis. Although PLE is usually fairly mild, it can be very irritating.)

"Since I got lupus, sun exposure in general gave me all sorts of problems with weird things happening to my skin," said Tania. "So, for awhile (during the treatments) I felt good on the inside, but not on the outside."

Tania needed to stop working a few years ago and today lives with her mother, but she's holding her own, she declared. "I've got a lot of joint pain, but I'm dealing with it."

"But this fatigue thing," she added, "this fatigue thing is getting on my nerves."

At this writing, Tania is one of the 54 total lupus cases McGrath has treated with UVA1. Some 70 percent have reported improvement while in therapy. Among the longest in therapy, about 13 years, is Lynn.

Also reached by phone at her New Orleans-area home, this 48-year-old Caucasian with a self-described "pretty fair complexion," said she began using UVA1 light "shortly after being diagnosed with lupus."

"My sons were 4 and 7 at the time. I was a stay at home mom, but I went back to school," she explained. "During my first term, my feet started hurting. I got a rash all over — over my whole body. My joints were just on fire. I had fevers. Everything was swollen. I felt like a sausage."

"My energy was non-existent. My kids would wake me up, I'd make them breakfast and go back to bed. They'd wake me up for lunch, make that, and go back to bed," said Lynn. "I couldn't even empty my dishwasher all at one time. I'd put away the glasses, then sit down. Put away the dishes, then sit down."

Not having health insurance at the time, Lynn needed to rely on the free health care services available through her school. They put her in touch with McGrath. In 1991, after a battery of tests to confirm her diagnosis, Lynn joined his study. "At first, the treatments were five days in a row for three weeks. After the second week, I was a new person. It was incredible."

"I remember I did three errands in a row on one day. I was amazed I could do it," she exclaimed. "Before, I'd do one, then go home and lay down."

Lynn stayed in the study for 7 years before acquiring her own 12-lamp sun canopy outfitted with TL/10R bulbs and UVA1 filter. "I bought it about 6 years ago from another patient who simply said she didn't need it anymore," Lynn explained. "I do it once every two weeks now for 40 minutes, 20 minutes per side."

Although she does sometimes experience "a little stiffness" in her hands first thing in the morning which "quickly goes away, other than that, my symptoms are gone," she said.

"I think it's had a cumulative effect over the years. My symptoms didn't all disappear during the first year, other than the fatigue."

In addition to her fatigue, rashes, and joint pain, Lynn also claims improvement in cognitive function. "There were times I just couldn't think. I knew what I wanted to say, I could picture it, but I couldn't get the word out. I'd be thinking 'bedspread,' but I just couldn't get the word out," she said. "Some days were better than others. Now that rarely, if ever, happens to me."

I asked, if after 13 years of regular exposures, she had much of a tan.

"I have a very slight sun tan," replied the blond-haired, blued-eyed Lynn. "But I do have a lot of age spots. Hundreds of them. They look like freckles."

What Lynn called "age spots" are also called "liver spots" and "lentigos," flat brown or black in color, they usually occur on the most sun-exposed areas of the body — backs of the hands, on the forearms, shoulders, face, and forehead. Common after age 40, the only possible complication is emotional distress. You know, like teenage pimples of youth.

"I'd probably have several anyway," Lynn surmised, "but I probably have more because of the light." After the lentigos began to appear, "I didn't like how it looked, so I now cover the upper part of my chest and my face."

"But it's worth it," she added quickly, "because I have a life."

"I'm just so happy to have my relationships back. In the beginning, everything changed. My husband was so worried about me, he had insomnia. Today, we don't even talk about my disease anymore," said Lynn. "It's no longer a problem. I think I'm in total remission."

"Have you thought about stopping the treatments then?" I asked.

"I've been thinking of stopping completely, but I'm a little hesitant to do that," she said. "I skipped three weeks once, while on vacation, and had no problem. But I gave myself an extra treatment before I left."

While not looking forward to the prospect of taking artificial sun baths for 13 years as Lynn has done, given how I used to feel, the prospect can also seem delightful. If or when I ever felt the disease was in full remission, I'd certainly stop long enough to check it out. Although it would be tough pulling the plug. Feeling well can be a powerful addiction.

DRUG-INDUCED LUPUS

Mentioned previously, drug-induced lupus requires medical treatment to identify and discontinue the offending medication. This is a partial list of drugs thought capable of causing lupus.

- Atenolol (Tenormin)
- Captopril (Capoten)
- Carbamazepine
- Chlorpromazine HCl (Thorazine)
- Clonidine HCl (Catapres)
- Danazol (Danocrine)
- Diclofenac (Cataflam, Voltaren)
- Ethosuximide (Zarontin)
- Gold compounds
- Griseofulvin
- Hydralazine HCl (Apresoline)
- Ibuprofen
- Interferon alfa
- Isoniazid (Laniazid, Nydrazid)
- Labetalol HCl (Normodyne, Trandate)
- Leuprolide acetate (Lupron)
- Levodopa (Dopar, Larodopa)
- Lithium carbonate
- Lovastatin (Mevacor)
- Mephenytoin (Mesantoin)
- Methyldopa (Aldomet)
- Methysergide maleate (Sansert)
- Minoxidil (Loniten, Rogaine)
- Nalidixic acid (NegGram)
- Nitrofurantoin (Furadantin, Macrobid, Macrodantin)
- Oral contraceptives
- Penicillamine (Cuprimine, Depen)
- Penicillin
- Phenelzine sulfate (Nardil)
- Phenytoin sodium (Dilantin)
- Prazosin (Minipress)
- Primidone (Mysoline)
- Procainamide HCl (Procan, Pronestyl)
- Promethazine HCl (Anergan, Phenergan)
- Propylthiouracil
- Psoralen
- Quinidine
- Spironolactone (Aldactone)
- Streptomycin sulfate
- Sulindac (Clinoril)
- Sulfasalazine (Azulfidine)
- Tetracycline
- Thioridazine HCl (Mellaril)
- Timolol maleate (Betimol, Timoptic)
- Tolazamide (Tolinase)
- Tolmetin sodium (Tolectin)
- Trimethadione (Tridione)

CHAPTER 3

BUSINESS IN THE CITY

D r. Hugh McGrath, Jr. is sitting in the back room of the Carnegie Deli at 854 7th Avenue. His eyes open wide as the waiter drops our large order on the small table between us.

"That's a sandwich?" he asks. "Looks like the entire cow."

At $17.95, the "Jumbo Corned Beef" could feed four. But after a long, hectic day on our feet and with little time for lunch, we hastily devour the thing and proceed to knock off half a bowl of pickles.

What brought us to Manhattan — me as a reporter and McGrath as a participant — was the 7th International Congress on SLE and Related Conditions, a professional medical conference held May 9-13, 2004. Along with a separate, parallel meeting held for patients, the 5th International Patient Congress, it drew about 1,500 lupus researchers, physicians and patients from around the world. Due to heightened security concerns and the new found difficulty of getting into the country, that was about half of what organizers originally expected.

We shared our day along with the sandwich and the sandwich proved more interesting. The day was filled with meeting people who never heard of UVA1, let alone cared about its potential as a lupus treatment.

While back in Chicago, given how much better I felt, I couldn't understand why this simple method was not flourishing. With a discouraging lack of available treatment options it didn't make much sense that the "lupus community" wasn't supporting, at the very least, further research. Even if the only effect UVA1 actually had was to alleviate fatigue, it could provide a phenomenal improvement for countless lives. A point a lupus researcher might miss, but a patient can't.

The few references to McGrath's research I found on various lupus websites all seemed to downplay the proven benefits and stress the potential risks. Caution was understandable, I reasoned, but the pessimism was not. When it came to balancing benefits against risks, McGrath had some impressive long-term data: He treated one group of 6 patients for nearly 3 1/2 years, and a few more for as long as 7 years, with no apparent toxic effects. In contrast, most therapeutic drugs get studied for only 6 weeks to 6 months before earning FDA approval. One reason we get warnings and drug recalls.

After running across an announcement online for the New York lupus congress, I called the event's chairman, Robert Lahita, M.D., Ph.D., listed in the event's program guide as Vice President and Chairman of Medicine at The Jersey City Medical Center. I told him my story and he seemed genuinely amazed.

I asked Lahita, one of the foremost lupus experts in the country (and as at it turned out, a very nice guy) why McGrath's work, after having been duly published in all the relevant top journals, had been largely ignored. Lahita said he remembered hearing about it, but was advised to overlook the findings because UVA light, along with UVB, is associated with skin cancer.

When I explained the UVA wavelength range that McGrath uses is thought by UV experts to be qualitatively different, and is now used successfully to treat severe atopic dermatitis at much higher doses than required for lupus, Lahita admitted to not knowing there might be a difference between UVA and UVA1.

He encouraged me to ask McGrath to submit an abstract of his latest work and attend the New York meeting. It took some convincing, but McGrath finally agreed to go. He submitted an abstract reporting two recent case studies showing UVA1's effectiveness in reversal of cognitive dysfunction and lowering anticardiolipin antibody levels. The latter never having been achieved in a patient before using any other agent, including drugs. [See Appendix B.]

McGrath's abstract was of course accepted, but since the roster of symposia speakers had already been set he was given a slot in what is called a "poster session" — a common event at medical and other meetings where a researcher presents their study results as a visual display, usually a poster board, which can include a brief narrative, tables, graphs, pictures, etc. The researcher then stands by the poster during an assigned time, usually for two hours while others walk around, take a look and ask questions. That's the theory.

Due to either poor planning, or with just too much else to do in New York, the few people who did show up for the poster sessions I attended (and I attended all of them) were the poster participants themselves. Most of them left after about 45 minutes because of the poor attendance. Which was understandable. The area set aside for the event was off the beaten path, and the windowless room lacked air-conditioning (it was fairly hot and humid that week in Manhattan). Perhaps more importantly, the physicians registered for the congress didn't receive continuing education credits for attending poster sessions as they did for the regular symposia. As one disgruntled poster participant remarked, "An open bar and a bowl of pretzels would have helped."

After registering for the congress early the first morning and stringing press credentials around my neck, I introduced myself to one of the event's vice-chairs, who also seemed to be the administrator responsible for the makeshift press room. I told her of my intention to do a story on McGrath's UVA1 treatment, and asked what she thought of it. "You don't want my opinion on that," she declared. When I answered I certainly did, she asked why I was writing down what she said.

"Because I'm a reporter," I replied. "I didn't say you could quote me," she returned. "You better not use my name."

I assured her she would remain anonymous, then thought it wise to change the subject. Not having had my morning coffee yet, I was a bit single-minded, however. "Do you know if there's any coffee in the press room," I asked. "You can buy your own coffee," she barked, before walking off.

That encounter generally mirrored the rest of the week. Every morning I bought my own coffee and most people had nothing to say — no one had ever heard of UVA1. Whenever I brought the subject up I was usually interrupted with this question: "But don't you know ultraviolet causes lupus flares?"

For those who had heard of UVA1 the verdict was already in. And it wasn't good. The therapy, it seemed, was getting nothing but bad press.

For example, among the books for sale in the congress's exhibit area was one edited by Lahita — the fourth edition of *Systemic Lupus Erythematosus* (Elsevier Academic Press, April, 2004), something of a bible in the field.

In Chapter 48, "Unproven and Experimental Therapies," UVA1 gets a brief mention: "The use of UVA1 light therapy for SLE, as counter-intuitive as it may seem, has been proposed based on specific immunomodulatory properties of electromagnetic waves in the 340-400nm" range.

The author concludes: "Modest effect sizes, technological details, and cost of the treatment have tempered enthusiasm for this therapy."

"Modest effect sizes" I assumed (and McGrath agreed) means the research to date has not shown UVA1 to affect kidney dysfunction. That could and should be resolved with further research. McGrath thinks the therapy might help with kidney inflammation as well.

As for "technological details," it's not rocket science. I built by myself a UVA1 light appliance that works quite well.

As for "cost," granted, medical devices capable of emitting UVA1 can be had in Europe for between $19,000 and $80,000 retail. A bit steep. Call it Yankee ingenuity, but using European parts I paid $5,000 for an appliance that does essentially the same thing. Based upon my research into getting the filters mass produced in the U.S., the total cost could at the very least be cut in half — meaning, $2,500 maximum for a therapeutically effective UVA1 light appliance. My point: It's the "tempered enthusiasm," or lack of demand, not the cost of the technology that should be considered a limiting factor.

Another published example picked up at the lupus congress that suggests how maligned this treatment is, was in the Spring 2004 issue of *Lupus Now*, a quarterly magazine published by the Lupus Foundation of America, Inc. In a section called "Ask the Experts," a patient writes: "Is the use of tanning beds okay for people with lupus?" In the course of answering "No," Richard D. Sontheimer, M.D., a member of the foundation's Medical/Scientific Advisory Council, referred to McGrath's work when he wrote: "Some research suggests that very long ultraviolet light wavelengths, in what is called the 'UVA1' range, can improve certain forms of lupus skin disease and mild forms of systemic lupus."

"This research has been somewhat controversial," Sontheimer continues, "because other research has found that higher doses of the same UVA1 wavelengths are capable of aggravating the systemic manifestations of lupus."

McGrath had no any idea what "other research" Sontheimer was referring to. Neither did Urbach: "I know of no evidence for that," he said. I contacted Sontheimer's office for the previously unreferenced study [Lupus, 1993 Aug; 2(4):247-50].

It turns out if you define "aggravating the systemic manifestations of lupus" to mean a lowly sun burn in some of the patients exposed, then Sontheimer's statement is technically correct. And if you allow "higher doses" to mean radiation levels about 60 times more intense than used in lupus treatments to cause those sun burns, he's also technically correct. But it's easy to be technically correct when you define your own terms. Sontheimer's assessment, I think, is both unfair and misleading.

Instead of exposing skin to the entire UVA1 spectrum as during a lupus treatment, the researchers Sontheimer cites, administered very high doses of specific single wavelengths — 320 nm (which is actually UVA2/UVB), 345 nm, 360 nm, and 375 nm — to cause the burns.

Although these researchers did not also test wavelengths in the visual range (400 nm to 700 nm), "Had they done so, I suspect that visible light at the greatly increased individual wavelength intensities or dose they were testing would have produced" a sun burn as well, said McGrath.

"Why did they not irradiate with broad spectrum UVA1? — or did they, and when finding nothing to report decided to irradiate in such a manner as to support a reason for publishing their data?" McGrath added. "What would have been surprising is if these massive doses of individual wavelengths failed to cause prolonged erythema in lupus patients...Lupus patients do not tolerate stress."

When Sontheimer wrote me to cite the study, he also cited another reason he wasn't a big fan of McGrath's research: "As an example of the potential clinical impact of these issues, I have been asked by LE patients based on Dr. McGrath's work if sunbathing or tanning after using a broad spectrum sunscreen might be therapeutic rather than risky. My response has been that this could be very risky and should be avoided until we know more about the effects of various doses of UVA1 on cutaneous LE and systemic LE disease activity."

McGrath's response to that critique was equally ardent: "As far as patients asking about suntanning with UVA or with sunscreens, the implication is that if patients misunderstand what the studies are reporting, the data should not have been reported. I cannot agree — it's hardly necessary to point to where that rationale would take us."

Equally disappointing as the published misinformation about UVA1 found in New York, was the lack of news about any other significant advance in possible treatments. However, there was one report about a new drug called Prestara (a patentable knock-off of DHEA) by Genelabs Technology Inc., that might be useful to counteract side effects of a current drug treatment. Sort of like putting a band-aid on a band-aid I thought.

(*News Update, October 6, 2004:* The band-aid fell off. Genelabs Technologies, Inc. stock plummeted after the company said its Prestara lupus drug failed in a clinical trial to meet its primary goal — increase the bone mineral density of women with SLE receiving glucocorticoids.)

Despite disappointment, it was not a wasted trip. I made my first lamentable, yet necessary visit to "Ground Zero." And there was that melt-in-your-mouth corned beef. During a patient lecture I also discovered, for me at least, a few interesting new facts. One such lupus factoid literally made me choke. This memorable event also involved a sandwich.

On the first day of the congress the organizers held a noon press conference to announce the establishment of "World Lupus Day." Box lunches were provided for reporters. I grabbed one marked "turkey/cheese," before leaving to attend a patient program called "Complementary/Alternative Therapies and Nutrition" (it turned out the lecturer hadn't heard of UVA1 either). Taking a seat in the empty back row, I stashed the lunch box under my chair and forgot about it until she started talking about nutrition. Then, I got hungry.

I squeezed a little mustard on the whole wheat bread covering the sandwich's contents, which included alfalfa sprouts along with the cheese. "Nice touch," I thought. I was about to eat the second half when the lecturer noted how alfalfa sprouts were known to cause flares. "Nice planning," I muttered, after spitting it back into the box. Apparently, no one imagined a reporter with lupus would have the strength to show up and cover the event. Then again, no one heard of UVA1.

I left New York with a better sense why McGrath's work hasn't made much of an impact. Not the least of which is the fact that medical meetings such as Lupus 2004 are primarily funded by pharmaceutical companies. Not unless say, the "Lamp Section" of the "National Electrical Manufacturers Association" gets into the act, would McGrath ever receive the welcome mat I think he deserves.

According to one lupus specialist, perhaps the most important reason McGrath's work is largely unknown is because many SLE researchers just don't read. I picked up on that possibility during the congress's "Gala Dinner."

The way the prominent M.D. I sat next to during dinner explained it, the total universe of active lupus researchers is relatively small, and they generally know what everyone else is doing.

"Sort of an inbred group," I ventured.

"Exactly," he said.

Consequently, there isn't much need to read the lupus-related journals since most already know the results long before any study gets published. Research such as McGrath's falls through the cracks.

I asked Urbach if he thought that was really the problem; if either a lack of time or inclination to thoroughly review all published research was keeping the UVA1 treatment option down.

"Most of these people have blinders on," said Urbach. "That's the problem."

A BRIEF, UNOFFICIAL HISTORY
OF SYSTEMIC LUPUS ERYTHEMATOSUS

400 BC — Hippocrates documents red ulcerating skin lesions which may or may not be connected with lupus.

About 1400 AD — The word lupus - Latin for wolf - is first used in a medical context to describe red ulcerations on the face.

1808 — Dr. Robert Willan, considered the founder of British dermatology, includes lupus in his formal classification of skin diseases. His description of lupus emphasized the disease's destructive nature and lack of any available treatment. He was, however, likely describing tuberculosis of the skin, still known as lupus vulgaris.

1851 — Pierre Louis Alphée Cazenave, a student of French dermatologist Blett, introduces the term lupus erythematosus and confirms this disease is distinct from other ulcerating skin disorders.

1875 — Dr. M. Kaposi, a Viennese dermatologist, is the first to recognize the systemic nature of lupus erythematosus and is the first to describe the butterfly rash.

1885-1904 — Dr. William Osler greatly expands upon the concept of SLE and describes in a series of papers the heart, lung, joint, brain, kidney and stomach symptoms. He also recognizes that some cases occur without skin involvement.

1948 — Dr. Malcolm Hargraves, a Mayo Clinic hematologist, discovers the LE cell and it quickly becomes the basis for diagnosing SLE. The discovery is the first clear sign that SLE could be an autoimmune disorder.

1950s — Anti-nuclear antibody tests (ANA) are first developed. Treatment with antimalarials begins in 1951. In 1952 corticosteroids are developed and used along with other immunosuppressives for the first time.

1959 — Researchers at the Otago Medical School discover New Zealand Brown x New Zealand White hybrid mice develop a lethal kidney disease that closely resembles lupus nephritis - the kidney disease which some SLE patients develop. This mouse has been studied in laboratories around the world. Other mice which develop lupus-like diseases have also been bred, particularly in the U.S.

1960s — The prognosis for lupus sufferers improves dramatically as diagnostic abilities improve, drugs are used more sensitively and public awareness begins to grow.

1990s — Dr. Hugh McGrath, Jr. pioneers the medicinal use of UVA1 light.

CHAPTER 4
DR. HUGH MCGRATH, JR.
ON UVA1 PHOTOTHERAPY

The intended format of this chapter was the time honored Q&A. I posed written questions, McGrath provided written answers. His responses were so far ranging and required such clarification, instead of publishing the questions I've come up with broad subject headings to introduce and help organize his thoughts. Ask a passionate research scientist a question, expect a complex answer.

ON EXPERIMENTING WITH
ULTRAVIOLET LIGHT IN LUPUS MICE:

My interest in the effects of ultraviolet light in lupus was triggered by the unusual adverse reactions of lupus patients to sunlight, in particular to the ultraviolet wavelengths emitted from the sun. Patients responded in a highly adverse manner to the shorter ultraviolet wavelengths, but curiously, seemed to have little problem with exposure to the longer ultraviolet wavelengths. Noonday sun, which contains the highest levels of the shorter wavelengths, is noxious to all people but is disease activating in lupus patients. Unlike a spate of dermatologic disorders triggered or augmented by sunlight, in lupus sunlight damages not only the skin but the internal organs as well. Their 'photosensitivity' is systemic, meaning throughout the system. This effect of the ultraviolet light in sunlight is unique to lupus. As lupus works primarily through the immune system, I decided to observe the effects of ultraviolet light on immune cells *in vitro*, which means isolated and placed in a Petri dish. While at the University of Virginia from 1977 to 1980 I found that very low doses of short wavelength ultraviolet light delivered to immune cells (lymphocytes) increases immune reactivity, a change that might be harmless or even beneficial in normal subjects, but could be harmful in patients already suffering from an overcharged immune system.

After arriving at Louisiana State University Health Sciences Center in 1980, I worked with a mouse model of lupus, known as the B/W mouse. The females of this species develop lupus spontaneously. Studies had shown that in this mouse, as in humans with lupus, short wavelength ultraviolet radiation (ultraviolet B) worsens disease. Remembering that patients with lupus had no significant problems with the longer wavelengths, known as ultraviolet A, I exposed half of a group of these mice to low doses (3.5 Joules/cm^2) of ultraviolet A radiation daily, leaving the other half of the group unexposed. Surprisingly, as the mice that were unexposed to UVA radiation died at the usual rate for these mice, those that were exposed to the UVA radiation lived on. After approximately half of the untreated mice and none of the treated mice had died, we sacrificed all the mice to determine what underlay this difference in mortality. We found that the UVA-irradiated mice had smaller spleens, lower levels of antibodies, and more normally acting immune cells than the non-irradiated mice. Although we had expected that the longer wavelengths would not bother lupus mice, we did not expect these wavelength exposures to diminish lupus activity and prolong survival.

ON UV WAVELENGTHS AND THE SKIN:

First, here's some photo physics that might interest you. Fluorescent lamps emit at the single wavelength of 254 nm which is in the UVC range, but this emission is absorbed by a phosphor that coats the glass tube and is re-emitted at longer wavelengths primarily in the visible range. What little UVB emissions exist are almost completely absorbed by the standard acrylic diffusers used almost universally to cover the fluorescent bulbs. What is emitted through these acrylic diffusers is essentially the same range of visible wavelengths emitted by the sun.

UVA bulbs, presently known as black light bulbs, emit at 325 nm to 440 nm, peaking at 360 nm. They are used to treat psoriasis. The sun lamps often used at tanning parlors emit wavelengths from 260 nm to 400 nm, peaking at 320 nm. The glass envelope in the sun lamp prevents escape of emissions shorter than 320 nm.

Sunlight emits its wavelengths in a somewhat bell-shaped curve starting at 300 nm and peaking at about 550 nm and then dropping down almost as quickly to about 950 nm, after which the curve flattens out beyond 1000 nm. The wavelengths between 400 nm and 700 nm are in the so-called photopic vision region — a region forming a bell-shaped curve that peaks at 550 nm. This curve incorporates the visible wavelengths that are essentially the same wavelengths emitted from commercial fluorescent lamps.

The skin is a protective organ acting as a barrier between adverse influences of the external environment and the internal milieu of the body. It processes influences of the external environment, most notably the sun, into actions that benefit the organism. The transformation within the skin of pre-Vitamin D3 to Vitamin D3 is a prime example. UVA1 irradiation is a defined range of ultraviolet wavelengths present in sunlight that have proven to be favorable to patients with lupus, despite the known adverse actions of other wavelength bands, most notably UVB.

There is a dynamism that has been established through the eons between terrestrial wavelengths and life on earth. Different wavelengths have different properties but as they always act in unison, the effects of these wavelengths are consistent and predictable. All of these wavelengths together comprise a balanced dynamism into which man has been integrated during his time on earth. Omitting one part of the sun's spectrum in favor of another cannot but create an entirely new biologic impetus. Effects that are not normally produced, perhaps never having been produced by this age-old agent, are unpredictable. They could be harmful. On the other hand, they might be helpful in a disease setting in which one disease aberrancy can compensate for another, especially if the aberrancies are both sunlight-related. Today, this type of interaction can and should be exploited if it leads to a beneficial effect.

Among the most critical differences in UV wavelengths on the skin are penetrance and energy. The shorter the wavelengths the less the penetrance. UVC barely penetrates the skin, UVB traverses the outer layer known as the epidermis, and UVA penetrates all the way down to the blood vessels. The greater penetration of UVA means that it affects deeper structures, such as blood vessels, far more than do the shorter wavelengths. With regard to energy, the longer wavelengths are less energetic than the shorter wavelengths, often making them less damaging. Additionally, the longer wavelengths are absorbed by different molecules, that is, by different cellular and extracellular constituents than are the shorter wavelengths.

A principle of photophysics states that for a substance to be acted upon by a particular wavelength it must absorb that wavelength. Chemical changes will occur only if a wavelength is absorbed. If a particular substance is transparent to that wavelength, the wavelength will have no effect. DNA, for example, can absorb UVB but not UVA wavelengths. Therefore, UVB but not UVA can damage DNA. UVB-induced damage is an important pathway of UVB disease activation in lupus. Few of the substances that absorb wavelengths in the UVA and UVA1 range have been identified. It is important that they are because it is by causing chemical changes in these substances that UVA1 photons work.

The balance that exists in the wavelengths from the sun that reach the earth explain why individual wavelength bands, such as A, B, C, A1 or A2, or even individual wavelengths, may have actions that cannot be reproduced during exposure to the entire spectrum of wavelengths. For example, UVB radiation causes suppression of the cellular immune system whereas UVA enhances it. Acting together the two may neutralize each another to some extent so there is less sum effect. Likewise, if one wavelength causes an action, another wavelength may prevent or even reverse that action.

ON EXPERIMENTING WITH
ULTRAVIOLET LIGHT IN LUPUS PATIENTS:

Following the mouse studies we irradiated lupus patients. In an open clinical trial we irradiated patients 5 days a week for three consecutive weeks with 6 J/cm^2/day of UVA1 irradiation. TL/10R lamps that emit ultraviolet radiation that is predominantly UVA1, with only 0.06 percent UVB and 0.03 percent UVA2 wavelengths, were obtained from the Philips company in The Netherlands. Patients tolerated this radiation well. Fatigue, joint pain, fever, malaise, and morning stiffness improved significantly, encouraging us to step up to a blinded, placebo-controlled study.

To improve on the TL/10R emissions, Mutzhas's UVASUN filters were obtained. These filters eliminate all the UVB and UVA2 radiation, which results in ultraviolet emissions that are 100 percent UVA1. This was done to avoid any dampening of the full effect of UVA1 radiation. Using this lamp/filter combination, a double-blind, placebo-controlled study enrolling 26 women to be irradiated over 18 weeks brought favorable results. The patients exposed to UVA1 radiation improved markedly over six weeks whereas patients exposed to visible light did not. All patients were then exposed to UVA1 for a further 12 weeks and improvement continued to the end. The amount of UVA1 that was needed for a beneficial response was about 6 J/cm^2/day, or about 1/6 of the amount needed to produce slight pinkness in the average Caucasian.

Six patients were selected for long-term treatment. They continued with one to two treatments per week for an average of 3.4 years. They maintained or even slightly improved upon the gains made during the initial 18 weeks. This study showed that long-term irradiation brought continued response.

Together these two studies indicated that low levels of UVA1 photons delivered to the skin in patients with lupus, effectively, comfortably, and progressively, relieved constitutional and other signs and symptoms of disease activity and reduced the need for medication.

HOW AND WHY UVA1 MIGHT WORK:

It is reasonable to assume that much or most of the ameliorative action of UVA1 irradiation is mediated through the skin, the most massive organ in the body and the primary target of the therapy. Characterized by widespread heightened immune disruption within the dermal-epidermal junction that lies just below the surface of the skin, the skin in lupus has the potential to contribute to the blood a generous overflow of inflammatory constituents capable of increasing overall disease activity. There are a number of mechanisms that might be contributing to this benefit. First of all, UVB irradiation causes movement of proteins from the nucleus of the cell to the cell surface where, in lupus, they can be bound by lupus antibodies that can destroy the cell. In contrast, UVA wavelengths not only fail to move these proteins from the nucleus to the cell surface but appear to inhibit this action caused by UVB as well as other agents, such as estrogens and viruses. UVA1 wavelengths may also help in lupus by a direct action on DNA. Accordingly, UVB damages DNA and UVA1 repairs it.

There are certain proteins in the cell that transmit signals from the environment, from the sun for example, to the nucleus. As an example, a protein called YAP-1 when acted upon by UVA1 irradiation, activates 70 different genes. The purpose of YAP-1 is to signal the nucleus that the cell is being irradiated by UVA1, so that the nucleus can respond appropriately. UVA1 irradiation releases singlet oxygen, a substance that causes repercussions, both good and bad, in the cell. The purpose of YAP-1 is to signal the nucleus so that the nucleus can release genes that sort out the responses to singlet oxygen, promoting those that are beneficial and inhibiting those that are not.

Accordingly, giving UVA1 irradiation is in effect like giving a medication which causes only certain genes to express their actions. This is helpful either because these genes are under expressed in lupus or their UVA1-induced increased expression compensates for a deficit in the disease. It is only recently in man's history and due to photo technological advances that it has become possible to irradiate people with only some of the wavelengths coming from the sun, each of these wavelengths or bands of wavelengths having different actions on the cell, its nucleus, and the body as a whole, and thereby able to control physiological responses. The technology has created an artificial system whose potential is desirable medicinally. The artificial system, especially following the recent isolation of the UVA1 wavelengths, appears particularly adapted to correcting aberrations in lupus, a complex disease that requires the activation of certain genes in certain cells to make those cells behave normally.

For the first time in history, groups of wavelengths and even individual wavelengths can be isolated and used to produce effects in a patient different from those produced by any other wavelength and often markedly different than the effects produced by all the wavelengths delivered together during natural sun exposure. The beneficial and harmful effects are being dissected. As the beneficial and harmful effects for lupus patients differ from the beneficial and harmful effects for those without lupus, this age-old source of energy has been broken down with special filters and delivered in the wavelengths that accord to the needs of the lupus patient.

As opposed to treating patients with synthetic medication that will likely be entirely foreign to the patient, UVA1 irradiation has been part of man's environment since his beginnings and has no doubt guided his evolution. It is the abnormalities produced in some that makes sunlight unfriendly and necessitates the dissecting out of certain wavelengths or wavelength bands, leaving the sun's wavelengths that prove friendly and beneficial.

The primary mechanism by which UVA1 photons work involves a process called apoptosis. This is the name given to scheduled cell death.

When immune cells, for example, have finished the work for which they have been commissioned, such as producing antibodies, they lie down and die, so to speak. More specifically they self-disassemble and are then neatly carried away, intact, by other cells designed for that purpose. The process of self-disassembly is known as apoptosis. If it were not for apoptosis, cells would just keep reproducing and functioning when no longer needed or no longer effective. Immune cells that produce antibodies would keep on doing so even when there was no longer a need. That is what happens in lupus. The antibodies needlessly produced in great abundance do damage. In lupus there appears to be a lack of apoptotic machinery. When apoptosis fails, not only do antibodies do damage but because of the failure of programmed cell death another form of cell death known as necrosis ensues. Unlike apoptosis, in which cells and all of their constituents are neatly removed, necrosis releases all of these constituents into the blood stream. These constituents are in a sense poisonous and have to be removed.

Although necrosis occurs, for example, anytime a person falls and breaks a bone, the apparatus for removing these substances is engaged only briefly and is therefore well tolerated. However, in lupus there is a constant stream of constituents released because there is an energy failure in lupus and apoptosis is an energy-dependent process. Failing apoptosis, necrosis supervenes and becomes the rule rather than the exception. Instead of the relatively inefficient systems normally called upon to cleanse the body of the rare release of necrotic constituents, a more permanent and efficient system is required. Accordingly, a network of antibodies is established and put permanently into place to intercept the constant stream of necrotic constituents released from the cells in lupus patients. For a half century, these antibodies have been viewed as the cause rather than response to the underlying disease process in lupus. Antibodies, such as anti-DNA and anti-SSA, are not the problem. They are the body's response to the problem. The problem is a deficit in energy production that cripples apoptotic mechanisms and leads to necrosis, which requires the production of antibodies. These antibodies are simply doing their job cleaning up debris.

Thus, in effect, UVA1 irradiation delivers a special form of energy, photon energy, that compensates for the energy deficit in lupus that leads to a failure of apoptosis. It does this by generating singlet oxygen. UVA1 photons are the best known generators of singlet oxygen and singlet oxygen is the best known natural generator of apoptosis. Because the failure of apoptosis in SLE is due to a failure in the production of ATP [adenosine triphosphate production = an energy-rich compound used for all energy-requiring processes in the body] and reactive oxygen species, the generation of singlet oxygen offers a compensatory pathway of apoptosis. In contrast to necrosis that releases cellular constituents into blood and tissues, singlet oxygen-induced apoptosis has the potential for removing the cells neatly, averting their march to necrosis.

It is our working hypothesis that the UVA1 irradiation-induction of singlet oxygen fosters a supplanting of necrosis by apoptosis, averting the release of cellular constituents and the consequences of that release. The UVA1-induction of singlet oxygen is limited to the skin. However, the skin is the largest organ in the body, and perhaps the most consistently and heavily involved in SLE, as indicated by the ongoing simmering immunoreactivity in the dermal-epidermal junction just below the skin's surface. Diminishing the release and overflow into the blood stream of cellular constituents from this massive organ can be expected to dampen systemic activity.

At present, Plaquenil, prednisone, and Cytoxan, key medications for treating lupus patients, all promote apoptosis but are toxic. UVA1 irradiation-induced apoptosis represents a gentle means of compensating for both the energy deficit and antibody binding-induced failures of apoptosis in these patients.

The discordance and often antagonism between the actions of different bands of ultraviolet wavelengths coming from the sun explains why UVA1 irradiation often counters the disease-based abnormalities in lupus while UVB irradiation promotes them. An additional means by which UVB wavelengths can injure lupus patients is in the normal propensity of UVB to stimulate movement of proteins from the nucleus of the cell to its surface. This occurs in all people exposed to enough sun to cause sunburn. It is the beginning of a progression to apoptosis that is designed to remove the injured cells without necrosis. Unfortunately, in lupus there are circulating antibodies to these same proteins so that when the proteins reach the surface of the cell they are bound by these antibodies and the union damages the entire cell which goes on to necrose. It is not only sunlight that brings about this progression. Estrogens and viruses can also promote it so that any of these factors can promote necrosis. As opposed to UVB wavelengths, UVA1 photons not only fail to move these proteins to the surface of the cell but in addition have been shown to promote early apoptosis, gently removing these sun-injured cells intact before the proteins migrating from the nucleus can reach the surface of the cell.

Even viruses may play into the disease and into the response to UVA1 irradiation. Viral like structures have been described in kidney, joint and skin cells of lupus patients. The capacity of UVA1 irradiation to promote apoptosis would serve to capture the viruses within the intact cells containing them, avoiding necrosis that would release all the intracellular constituents allowing the viruses to disseminate and invade other cells.

ON THE TOXIC, BENEFICIAL AND OTHER EFFECTS OF UVA1 IRRADIATION, INCLUDING RECENT STUDY FINDINGS:

Occasionally, patients will develop pinkness, or even a mild sunburn from UVA1 irradiation. Otherwise, the adverse effects of UVA1 irradiation are negligible, such as an increased sensitivity of fair skinned patients to the development of harmless age spots or lentigos.

Patients taking drugs that cause photosensitivity will experience photosensitivity as much or even more with UVA1 than with shorter wavelengths such as UVB. Most drug photosensitivity is due to wavelengths in the UVA range, so we ask our patients to avoid the drugs associated with photosensitivity. The photosensitivity caused by drugs is entirely separate from lupus photosensitivity which is due, for the most part and most severely, to UVB radiation.

The most gratifying result of treatment for the majority of patients was reversal of the profound fatigue that characterizes lupus. The fatigue is like that of fibromyalgia, so we tested a group of six patients with fibromyalgia but without lupus. We found them essentially unresponsive to the UVA1 radiation therapy. Lupus patients can also have fibromyalgia and one of our lupus study patients who suffered from both disorders insisted that she could tell the difference between the fatigues. She reported that the UVA1 therapy helped only the fatigue due to her lupus.

We tested the action of UVA1 on a group of six patients with rheumatoid arthritis and found no improvement. This was not surprising.

Rheumatoid arthritis is a disorder that is mediated by immune cells that emit toxins, unlike lupus in which cells emit autoantibodies. On the other hand, three week exposures to UVB radiation that suppresses cellular immunity brought significant relief to a group of 26 rheumatoid arthritis patients. We have not pursued this study because long-term UVB irradiation is toxic.

UVA1 irradiation is unique. When delivered to the skin at these low levels it effectively, comfortably, progressively, and without apparent side effects, relieves constitutional and other signs and symptoms of disease activity. It reduces the need for medication and diminishes antibody levels. Although our working hypothesis is that these deeply penetrating photons bring about their benefits by suppressing inflammation within the skin, a massive organ that can contribute a considerable supply of irritating or damaging constituents overflowing into the bloodstream of lupus patients, the deeply penetrating UVA1 photons may also act directly on cells percolating through the skin at the time of irradiation. The action of this therapy is not mediated through the eyes as these are covered by opaque glasses throughout the therapeutic sessions. UVA1 irradiation is not only a new mode of therapy but it offers a new perspective on the complex role of ultraviolet light in lupus.

However, as with any new therapy there are theoretical dangers. One of these derives from the experience that long term exposure to other forms of ultraviolet radiation leads to the development of skin tumors. Although free of this risk to date, UVA1 and visible wavelengths have been implicated investigationally in the generation of melanoma. A certain genus of fish developed melanoma after a single exposure to individual wavelengths of UVA and visible light. Although the production of melanoma by delivering single wavelength of UVA1 or visible light seems surprising, the individual wavelengths were delivered at enormously high levels and without the balancing action of accompanying wavelengths. It is a markedly artificial system of exposure never experienced in nature or phototherapy. No tumor of any kind has ever been reported in association with UVA1 despite its use by dermatologists for skin diseases this past decade in much higher doses than those used for lupus. Nevertheless, all of our patients are instructed to check with a dermatologist once a year.

A group of investigators did irradiate patients with levels of UVA an order of magnitude higher than our UVA1 levels and inclusive of UVA2, the band now considered functionally an extension of UVB. This produced rashes as would be expected in patients sensitive to UVB and UVA2. Another research group reported that emissions from a photocopier produced a rash in a lupus patient and this, too, involved UVA2 emissions. In a third case investigators elicited rashes not only from UVA and UVA1, but even visible light when they irradiated patients with single wavelengths from these sources. When single wavelengths are used, there may be 10 to 100 times more of that wavelength than when it is delivered within an entire band, such as UVA. Moreover, the wavelengths in the ultraviolet spectrum are in balance and without the other wavelengths to buffer its action, the action of an isolated wavelength becomes uncontained and unpredictable. This type of procedure showed that a single UVA1 wavelength can cause redness in a patient with lupus. It is a meaningless observation.

Although joint pain, photosensitivity, skin rashes, mouth ulcers, headache, depression and insomnia respond to UVA1 therapy, the most gratifying response for the patient has been the loss of fatigue. This observation has heightened our own awareness of fatigue as a major source of disability in lupus. Moreover, along with the favorable responses to headache, depression and insomnia, it suggested that UVA1 irradiation may be dampening abnormal central nervous system disease activity.

We therefore tested two patients before and after treatment with PET scans to determine the effect of bodily UVA1 irradiation on the brain. In the first of these patients there was marked disruption indicated by the PET scan before treatment that paralleled the patient's difficulty with memory and concentration. These abnormalities disappeared completely over a period of months, as her concentration and fatigue improved. The second patient had brain damage due to the presence of anticardiolipin, an antibody often seen in lupus. During the six months of her UVA1 irradiation therapy the anticardiolipin antibody disappeared and the cognitive deficits stopped progressing both clinically and by PET scan even though the damage already sustained was permanent and irreversible.

We have not tested men adequately and we have not tested patients with renal disease adequately. We have no reason to believe, however, that this therapy would not be helpful in these cases as well.

Several treatment caveats apply: In spite of clinical improvement, the underlying disease persists and patients must continue to be monitored closely by their physicians. Patients need to obtain clearance from a dermatologist at least once annually. Exposures to UVA1 should never be prolonged or uncomfortable. Ongoing therapy is required for the action of UVA1 to persist. The changes in lupus are brought about through the skin and not the eyes which must always be covered. The promise of the observations made to date lie in the usefulness of UVA1 radiation in allowing patients to live with their disease, not in eliminating it.

These studies should contribute to a fuller understanding of disease pathogenesis tied as it is with its complex interrelationship with sunlight. Successful separation of the UV wavelength band has been key in determining the effectiveness of UVA1 irradiation as a therapeutic agent in lupus.

Lastly, I'd like to acknowledge the National Institutes of Health and the Tulane/LSU General Clinical Research Center, Charity Hospital, New Orleans, LA, for their continued support.

CHAPTER 5

WHAT'S NEXT?

Wish I knew. If I did this wouldn't be a one page chapter.

What happens next is largely up to you, the lupus patient.

If you would like to try the UVA1 light method, tell your doctors. Especially if they're associated with a research hospital or clinic. If they're not, ask anyway.

Ask them to consider becoming a part of McGrath's Phase II multi-center clinical trial. Explain to them how eager you are to join. And give them this book.

Don't assume your doctor will respond negatively to your request. Many have grown to acknowledge the effectiveness of certain non-drug approaches and are willing to take a serious look at whatever seems to work. For additional clinical trial information, they should contact McGrath directly:

Hugh McGrath, Jr., M.D.
Louisiana State University Medical School
1542 Tulane Avenue
New Orleans, LA 70112

504-568-4630

DR. NIELS
RYBERG FINSEN

In the course of my research I ran across the work of Dr. Niels Ryberg Finsen. I mentioned to Dr. Frederick Urbach how surprising it was to learn that one of the very first medical Nobels was awarded in 1903 to a man who treated with UV a disease called lupus vulgaris.

(For a biography of Finsen visit the Nobel Foundation's website — http://nobelprize.org/medicine/laureates/1903/finsen-bio.html)

Not only was I was struck by the similarity of name, but how 100 years ago the international medical community formally recognized the therapeutic value of UV, whether they knew how it worked or not. Urbach, an acknowledged pioneer in the field himself, had a story. "You know," he said causally, "I tested Finsen's original equipment."

For many years after Finsen's pioneering efforts, said Urbach, other researchers assumed he hit upon the therapeutic value of UVB. It was generally accepted early in this century that what's called UVA today had no biologic effects.

During his earliest research, "Finsen used sunlight, filtered through a large glass lens," Urbach explained. In the lens's center, he circulated a solution of copper sulfate in water to remove the sun's infrared wavelengths. Urbach got a hold of one of the original lenses from the research institute Finsen established in Europe, and as he expected, "virtually no UV wavelengths shorter than 320 nm passed through. It was all UVA," said Urbach, with some obvious satisfaction.

THE NOBEL PRIZE IN
PHYSIOLOGY OR MEDICINE 1903

Presentation Speech by Professor the Count K.A.H. Mörner,
Rector of the Royal Caroline Institute, on December 10, 1903

Your Majesty, Your Royal Highnesses, Ladies and Gentlemen.

This year's Nobel Prize for Physiology or Medicine has been awarded by the Council of Professors of the Caroline Institute to Professor Niels Finsen of Copenhagen in recognition of his work on the treatment of diseases, and in particular the treatment of lupus vulgaris by means of concentrated light rays.

Finsen's studies in connection with this disease constitute the most well-known and the most fruitful part of his work and are responsible for the important role played by phototherapy in medical art today. His first steps in the field of phototherapy, however, were directed towards general biological problems related to the effects of light on the organism. This led him to consider a number of specific problems concerning the effects of light on the skin in certain diseases. At first his research was not concerned with lupus but with another disease, smallpox. This first project in the field of therapeutics was certainly far removed from the principles that Finsen followed later in the treatment of lupus and other diseases, but it prepared the way none the less for his major research in this latter field.

In 1893 Finsen recommended the use of red light in the treatment of smallpox; this treatment, by protecting the skin against harmful light rays, was believed to facilitate the healing of the skin lesions and prevent the appearance of scars which are often the sequel to this disease. An analogous form of treatment for smallpox had in fact been in use many years before and had even been current during a part of the nineteenth century. A firm basis for this practice was lacking however. The situation was far more favourable when Finsen began his research on the subject. In 1889 Widmark's important work had demonstrated that the most refrangible rays of the spectrum, in particular the ultraviolet rays, had a strong and specific effect on those parts of the body surface which were exposed to them. This effect is quite different from the irritations or burnss produced by heat rays. At first no effect, or at the most a slight one, is apparent, but a few hours after exposure to the rays a certain degree of irritation is felt which progressively increases in intensity for about twenty-four hours and then gradually subsides. Finsen's proposed treatment of smallpox made use of Widmark's findings in this field. His method consisted in filtering off the ultraviolet rays by means of red glass and red curtains, etc., thus preventing their irritative effect on the affected skin, without having to keep the patient in total darkness.

Although this work brought recognition for Finsen, it is nevertheless of secondary importance when compared with the results of his further research. Finsen's stroke of genius in his later work was to attempt to make therapeutic use of the powerful biological effects of highly refrangible rays. In this way he blazed the trail for scientific phototherapy and for the curative use also of other rays than those contained in ordinary light.

Finsen's decision to follow this line of research was influenced by the phenomenon that light has the property of preventing the development of bacteria and even of killing micro-organisms. This phenomenon had already been observed in 1877 by Downes and Blunt and had been confirmed and studied by a number of scientists such as Duclaux, Roux, Buchner and others, on bacterial cultures, before Finsen undertook to apply it to living tissue containing bacteria. In this case also the active rays are the high-refraction rays of the spectrum. In considering the effects of light on living organisms containing bacteria, an explanation of the results obtained must take into account an essential factor other than the effect of light on pathogenic micro-organisms, namely, the already mentioned effects of light on the tissue itself. The question as to which of these two factors is most important in the therapeutic use of light will no doubt be the subject of further research. Whatever the answer may be to this question, the effective rays are the ones strongly refracted. The lower refraction rays, on the other hand, are of little use and, since they have the great disadvantage of producing combustion, must, as far as possible, be eliminated. Finsen's method is therefore in no way comparable to certain previous attempts to treat lupus by burning the affected tissue with a burning-glass.

The treatment of lupus by Finsen's method is carried out in the following way. Sunlight, or more frequently the light from a powerful electric-arc lamp (both forms containing a high proportion of active rays) is concentrated by means of lenses of appropriate composition into a beam from which the heat rays have been as far as possible eliminated; this beam is projected on a small area of affected skin, which has been drained of blood by pressure. The beam of light is applied continuously for one hour. Immediately afterwards the treated area becomes red and a little inflamed. During the next few days, this irritation of the skin increases, and then soon after begins to decrease and it is at this point that healing commences and scar tissue begins to form, which eventually produces a surface almost exactly like normal skin. Every part of the diseased area is treated consecutively, repeating the process twice on the same area if this proves necessary. This treatment has no unpleasant effects but it is expensive, requires constant supervision and considerable time. The results obtained, however, greatly outweigh these disadvantages. This method has proved of use in the treatment of a number of other skin diseases, but it has been particularly successful in the treatment of lupus vulgaris. None of the methods previously used for the treatment of this disease has produced results which can in any way be compared to those obtained with phototherapy.

Lupus vulgaris is, as we know, a form of tuberculosis, with localized lesions on the skin, especially that of the face, such as the nose, eyelids, lips and cheeks. The skin is gradually eroded, the face sometimes becomes dreadfully disfigured, and finally transforms patients into objects of repulsion. The chronic and progressive nature of this disease is particularly marked: it may remain active for ten years, twenty years, or even longer and, until now, it has proved resistant to all treatment. Even when patients had sufficient courage to persevere with these forms of treatment their hopes were dashed more often than not; rarely was a permanent improvement possible in this dreadful disease.

Thus it was that Finsen's method was hailed as a benefit to humanity when his treatment of lupus gave results which can without exaggeration be described as brilliant.

Finsen began to treat his first case of lupus in November 1895. Although the method had not yet been developed far, and although the case itself was of considerable severity, having proved resistant to all the current forms of treatment most energetically applied, the results were most satisfactory. News of this success soon spread: patients suffering from lupus left their hiding places and hurried from far and near to seek a cure or some relief from their suffering. They were rarely disappointed.

The new method soon obtained recognition from the medical world and became current practice. It also gained considerable support from philanthropists outside medical circles. The very next year, in 1896, the Finsen Institute of Phototherapy was founded in Copenhagen with funds obtained largely from generous private donations; the State and the City authorities also contributed. This Institute, devoted to research on the biological effects of light and the practical medical application of the results obtained, has since gradually been greatly developed and improved. It is now housed in its own recently equipped building, which includes a clinical section for the treatment of patients and an experimental research laboratory. It has a large staff including 8 doctors, 53 nurses, 3 assistants, other employees and numerous domestics.

Finsen's method for treating lupus is still used in the Institute. This year a report was published containing the cases of lupus treated during the first six years, up to and including November, 1901, in which 800 cases are described. The results are particularly satisfactory and are far superior to those obtained previously in the battle against this disease.

In 50 percent of these cases the skin disease was cured, although in many of them the lesions were extensive and of long standing. In a great number of cases, so much time has elapsed since the recovery that one considers this as permanent.

In the other 50 percent of these cases, in which a complete cure was not achieved, a partial cure or a considerable improvement was obtained in most cases. In only a very small number of cases, approximately 5 percent of all cases, treatment was unsuccessful or produced only temporary results. From the beginning of December 1901 until the end of October of this year, 300 further cases of lupus were treated. It has been noted that in recent years the proportion of cases of early lupus is much higher than before. As Finsen has said, it seems that in Denmark the time will soon come when the last chronic cases of lupus will have disappeared. Since cases of early lupus respond more easily to treatment, the future is most encouraging.

This method represents an immense step forward and the work of Professor Finsen has led to developments in a field of medicine which can never be forgotten in the history of medicine. For this reason he deserves the eternal gratitude of suffering humanity.

An illness, from which he has long suffered, unfortunately prevents Professor Finsen from being here today.

I therefore ask you, Count Sponneck, as representing Denmark, to accept on behalf of Professor Finsen the tribute which the Council of Professors of the Caroline Institute pays to your eminent fellow countryman in awarding him this year's Nobel Prize, and I am particularly happy to do so in the knowledge that this tribute has been won by a brother from over the Sund.

A P P E N D I X   B

RESEARCH REFERENCE

Lupus UVA1 Phototherapy Research,

1987-2003

ULTRAVIOLET-A LIGHT PROLONGS SURVIVAL AND IMPROVES IMMUNE FUNCTION IN (NEW ZEALAND BLACK x NEW ZEALAND WHITE)F$_1$ HYBRID MICE

HUGH McGRATH, Jr., ELIZABETH BAK,
and JOSEPH P. MICHALSKI

Source: Arthritis and Rheumatism, Vol. 30, No. 5, May 1987

© 1987 John Wiley & Son, Inc.

Although ultraviolet (UV) light is generally harmful to patients with systemic lupus erythematosus, most clinical and immunologic studies of UV exposure have evaluated the effects of UV-B (280-320 nm). The long-wavelength UV-A band (320-400 nm), however, is less toxic than UV-B and has different immunologic actions. Therefore, we studied the effect of UV-A irradiation on survival and immunologic function in the (New Zealand black x New Zealand white)F$_1$ hybrid mouse model of systemic lupus erythematosus. Twenty-one (New Zealand black x New Zealand white)F$_1$ mice were treated with 3.5 joules/cm^2/day of UV-A light for 5 days each week, beginning at age 10 weeks. A control group consisted of 20 untreated animals. All UV-A-irradiated mice survived to 32 weeks, compared with 12 of 20 mice in the nonirradiated group ($P = 0.0013$). Splenomegaly was significantly decreased in the irradiated mice ($P < 0.03$). Mice that received UV-A treatment combined with depilation had significantly improved lymphocyte responses to phytohemagglutinin and lipopolysaccharide and significantly decreased levels of anti-DNA antibodies compared with mice that received neither treatment. Reductions in spleen size and anti-DNA antibody titer were significantly correlated with improved parameters of lymphocyte function. These results suggest that a relatively small dose of UV-A exerts significant therapeutic action in murine lupus, perhaps through an effect on immunologic regulation.

Ultraviolet (UV) light is a well-documented contributory factor in the induction or exacerbation of systemic lupus erythematosus (SLE) (1). Most of the harmful effects of UV light have been attributed to UV-B, and it is primarily this band of wavelengths that is absorbed by DNA. UV-A (320-400 nm) is negligibly absorbed by DNA (2). Moreover, UV-A is far more abundant in terrestrial sunlight than is UV-B (3), and it penetrates the epidermis more effectively than does UV-B (4), and reaches the dermis with its circulating mononuclear cells. Although the effects of UV-A on immune function are not precisely understood, it may exert immunostimulatory action in experimental models in which UV-B is immunosuppressive (5,6).

We studied the effect of UV-A irradiation on survival, immunity, and autoimmunity in the (New Zealand black x New Zealand white)F_1 hybrid (NZB/NZW) mouse model of SLE. We report that long-term exposure to low-dose UV-A light prolongs the survival of NZB/NZW mice, while augmenting in vitro cellular immunologic function and decreasing autoantibody production.

MATERIALS AND METHODS

Animals. Forty-two female NZB/NZW mice were obtained from Jackson Laboratories (Bar Harbor, ME). They were fed ad libitum a commercial diet (Purina Laboratories, St. Louis, MO) plus tap water and were housed at 24°C with a daily 12-hour/12-hour fluorescent light/dark cycle.

Treatment protocol. A bank of 8 black-light lamps (F20T12-BL; Westinghouse, Bloomfield, NJ) that emit predominantly UV light of peak wavelength 355 was placed 30 cm above the animals. The irradiance was $1.3 \times 10^{-3} W/cm^2$, as measured with an SEE015 no. 1699 photodetector (International Light, Newburyport, MA), and <0.5% of the light emitted was UV-B, as measured by an SEE240 no. 1606 detector (International Light). Beginning at 10 weeks of age, mice received a dose of 3.5 joules (J)/cm^2 of UV-A irradiation 5 times per week for 22 weeks. Gentle air circulation during irradiation maintained a constant temperature, although heat emission was negligible.

The mice were divided into UV-A-irradiated and nonirradiated groups, and were subdivided according to the method used for the weekly removal of their dorsal hair: electric clippers or depilatory agent. The depilatory agent (Neet; Whitehall Laboratories, New York, NY) is a thioglycolic acid with a pH of 10-11. This material breaks disulfide bonds and removes hair at the skin level. Removal of hair with this agent may increase light penetration 10-15-fold compared with simple shaving (7). The 4 groups were as follows: group A (n = 10), irradiated and treated with the depilatory agent; group B (n = 11), irradiated and shaved; group C (n = 11), treated with depilatory agent; group D (n = 9), shaved (a tenth mouse originally assigned to this group escaped 1 week after the start of the study).

Deaths began to occur in the nonirradiated mice at 26 weeks of age. When the mice were age 32 weeks, the study was terminated because of a rapidly increasing mortality rate. The surviving mice were killed by cervical dislocation, and used for immunologic study. Immediately before killing, blood was obtained from the retroorbital plexus, and serum was separated for serologic studies. Spleens were removed using an aseptic technique, and the cells were teased from the stroma and isolated for mononuclear cell counts and in vitro functional studies.

Anti-double-stranded DNA (anti-dsDNA). Anti-dsDNA antibodies were assayed by the *Crithidia luciliae* technique, using a commercially available kit (Meloy, Springfield, VA). The manufacturer's instructions were followed, but were modified by the use of fluorescein isothiocyanate-conjugated goat F(ab)$_2$ anti-mouse IgG antibodies (Tago, Burlingame, CA).

Mitogen-stimulated lymphocyte proliferation and interleukin-2 (IL-2) production. Spleen cells (5 x 10^5) were cultured in 0.2-ml aliquots of RPMI 1640 supplemented with 10% heat-inactivated fetal calf serum, 1% glutamine, and 1% antibiotic/antimycotic, and buffered with 10 mM HEPES in the flat-bottomed wells of tissue culture plates (Costar, Cambridge, MA). Cultures were either unstimulated or had a final concentration of 20 µg/ml of lipopolysaccharide (LPS) or 1 µg/ml of phytohemagglutinin (PHA). After a 42-hour incubation with LPS (66 hours with PHA) at 37°C, cultures were pulsed with 1 μCi of tritiated thymidine (^{3}H-TdR), and they were harvested onto glass-fiber filters 6 hours later. The amount of incorporated ^{3}H-TdR was determined with a Beckman LS-250 scintillation counter (Beckman Instruments, Houston, TX).

Identical PHA-stimulated cultures were harvested at 24 hours and the supernatant assayed for IL-2, using a microassay with a murine IL-2-dependent cytotoxic T lymphocyte line (CTLL-2), as previously described (8).

Statistical analysis. Differences between the immune functions of the treatment groups were tested by the Mann-Whitney rank sum test, on a TI-59 programmable calculator (Texas Instruments, Lubbock, TX) using the applied statistics software module. Group survival was compared by Fisher's exact test, and correlations were made by linear regression analysis on a VAX 11780 (Digital, Maynard, MA).

RESULTS

Survival of female NZB/NZW mice treated with UV-A light. Twenty-one of the 41 NZB/NZW mice were treated with UV-A light 5 times per week from 10 weeks of age, as described in Materials and Methods. All of the irradiated mice survived to the end of the experiment. In contrast, the mice that were not treated with UV-A light developed ascites, and deaths began to occur when the animals were 26 weeks of age. A mortality curve similar to that previously reported for female mice of this strain (9) was seen. By age 32 weeks, 8 of 20 (40%) of the untreated mice had died, compared with none of the 21 treated animals (P = 0.0013 by Fisher's exact test).

Effect of UV-A light on splenomegaly. The total splenic mononuclear cell count, an indirect measure of splenomegaly, was significantly decreased in UV-A-irradiated animals compared with nonirradiated animals (P < 0.03).

Effect of UV-A light on splenic lymphocyte function. The PHA responses of group A mice (UV-A irradiation potentiated by depilation) were significantly higher (P < 0.04) than those of group D animals (neither UV-A nor depilation), whereas groups B and C, in which either the depilatory agent or UV-A was omitted, had intermediate responses.

Similarly, group A mice had a significantly higher mean LPS response than did group D animals ($P < 0.007$).

Effect of UV-A light on anti-DNA antibodies. Group A animals had a significantly lower geometric mean anti-dsDNA titer than did group D mice (1:46 versus 1:160, $P < 0.05$). As with lymphocyte responsiveness, mice that had been treated with either UV-A light alone or the depilatory agent alone had intermediate levels.

Correlations. Splenomegaly, measured by the splenic mononuclear cell count, was inversely correlated with the results of assays of lymphocyte function (PHA: $r = -0.48$, $P = 0.005$; LPS: $r = -0.44$, $P = 0.01$). Another measure of autoimmunity, the anti-DNA antibody titer, also had striking negative correlations with the proliferative responses to PHA ($r = -0.52$, $P = 0.002$) and to LPS ($r = -0.39$, $P = 0.03$).

DISCUSSION

Long-term intermittent exposure to UV-A light increased the survival of female NZB/NZW mice. The nonirradiated mice had a survival curve that was comparable with that previously described for this strain (9), with 40% of the mice dying by age 32 weeks. In contrast, none of the irradiated mice died during the same period. In addition, splenomegaly, a measure of autoimmunity (10), was significantly decreased in the irradiated animals.

Lymphocyte function, as measured by responsiveness to mitogens, was increased and anti-dsDNA antibody levels were decreased in the mice in which UV-A penetrance was enhanced by the use of a depilatory agent (group A), compared with those mice treated with neither agent (group D). Group B and group C animals, in which either the depilatory agent or the UV-A irradiation was omitted, had intermediate responses. Selection may have affected the results in groups C and D, since presumably, the sickest animals with the poorest lymphocyte responses and highest anti-dsDNA antibody titers would have died. The significant correlations of improved cellular immune function with decreased spleen size and levels of anti-dsDNA antibodies suggest that autoantibody production might be reduced through augmentation of cellular immune function.

An inverse relationship between mitogen responsiveness and disease activity in NZB/NZW mice has been reported previously (11). Mice of this strain exhibit vigorous immune responsiveness before the onset of disease (11), but become progressively less responsive to mitogens such as PHA and LPS as they age and develop evidence of autoimmunity (12,13). Therapeutic regimens that prolong survival, such as total lymph node irradiation (14) or administration of prostaglandin E_1 (15), androgens (16,17), or thymosin (18), are associated with a preservation of PHA responsiveness. Augmented responses to LPS have also been associated with successful therapy in NZB/NZW mice (19). In those studies, normalization of in vitro lymphocyte function was associated with decreased autoimmunity and, usually, with increased survival. One interpretation of the correlation between improved immune function and increased survival in mice in our study (as well as in others) is that autoimmune manifestations are improved by modulation of immune regulation.

Ultraviolet light has profound effects on the immune systems of normal mice. In most studies, investigators have used UV-B light, which has a variety of systemic suppressive effects, e.g., on the rejection of UV-induced tumors (20), on contact hypersensitivity (21), and on Ia expression on macrophages (22). The effects of UV-A light have received less attention and differ importantly from those of UV-B. UV-A light, for example, enhances systemic cell-mediated immunity, in contrast to the suppressive properties of UV-B (5). Likewise, UV-A light increases spleen cell DNA synthesis and release in vitro in NZB/NZW mice, whereas UV-B is inhibitory (6). These observations suggest that UV-A light has a less suppressive effect on the immune system than does UV-B and that, under some circumstances, UV-A may be immunostimulatory. An immunostimulatory effect of UV-A light may have contributed to the improved immunologic function and decreased autoimmunity in our treated NZB/NZW mice.

Most investigators studying the effects of UV light on NZB/NZW mice have used UV-B, and, in general, they have found it to be harmful. Our study animals, in contrast, had improved survival and improved immune function. The dosage of UV-A light we administered probably represents less than that absorbed during a 1-hour exposure to early morning or late afternoon sun, and about one-sixth the amount required to produce minimal erythema in normal humans. Thus, a relatively innocuous dose of an environmental agent to which nearly all of us are exposed on a regular basis may have profound salutary effects in a serious immunologic disease. A cautious trial of UV-A therapy in human subjects may be warranted.

ACKNOWLEDGEMENTS

We are grateful to Dr. Henry Jolly for his assistance, and to Dr. Robert Elston and Karl Cambre for their statistical expertise.

REFERENCES

1. Rothfield NF: systemic lupus erythematosus: clinical and laboratory aspects, Arthritis and Allied Conditions. Ninth edition. Edited by DJ McCarty. Philadelphia, Lea & Febiger, 1979, pp 691-714

2. Tan EM, Freeman RG, Stoughton RB: Action spectrum of ultraviolet light induced damage to nuclear DNA in vivo. J Invest Dermatol 55:439-443, 1970

3. Parrish JA, Anderson RR, Urbach F, Pitts D: Biological Effects of UV Radiation with Emphasis on Human Response to UV-A. New York, Plenum Press, 1978, p 74

4. Everett MA, Yeargers E, Sayre RM, Olson RL: Penetration of epidermis by ultraviolet rays. Photochem Photobiol 5:533-542, 1966

5. Morison WL: The effects of UVA radiation on immune function (abstract). Photochem Photobiol (suppl) 41:6s, 1985

6. Golan DT, Borel Y: Increased photosensitivity to near-ultraviolet light in murine SLE. J Immunol 132:705-710, 1984

7. Daynes RA, Bernard EJ, Gurish MF, Lynch DH: Experimental photoimmunology: immunologic ramifications of UV-induced carcinogens. J Invest Dermatol 77:77-85, 1981

8. Michalski JP, McCombs CC: Reduction of excessive background counts in an IL-2 microassay by incubation of indicator cells at 37ºC. J Immunol Methods 78:159-160, 1985

9. Dixon FJ: Murine lupus: a model for human autoimmunity. Arthritis Rheum 28:1081-1088, 1985

10. Theofilopoulos AN, Dixon FJ: Murine models of systemic lupus erythematosus. Adv Immunol 37:269-300, 1985

11. Talal N, Steinberg AD: Pathogenesis of autoimmunity in New Zealand black mice. Curr Top Microbiol Immunol 64:79-103, 1974

12. Raeder R, Freimer EH, Pansky B, Senitzer D: Response of peripheral blood lymphocytes from the (NZB/NZW) F_1 mouse to phytohemagglutinin. Clin Immunol Immunopathol 6:174-181, 1976

13. Keyes GG, Bickens RA, Kersey JH: Immunopathology of Sjogren-like disease in NZB/NZW mice. J Oral Pathol 6:288-295, 1977

14. Kotzin BL, Arndt R, Okada S, Ward R, Thach A, Strober S: Treatment of NZB/NZW mice with total lymphoid irradiation: long lasting suppression of disease without generalized immuno-suppression. J Immunol 136:3259-3265, 1986

15. Krakauer KA, Torrey SB, Zurier RB: Prostaglandin E_1 treatment of NZB/W mice. III. Preservation of spleen cell concentrations and mitogen induced proliferative responses. Clin Immunol Immunopathol 11:256-266, 1978

16. Dauphinée MJ, Kipper S, Roskos K, Wofsy D, Talal N: Androgen treatment of autoimmune NZB/W mice enhances IL-2 production (abstract). Arthritis Rheum (suppl) 24:S64, 1981

17. Michalski JP, McCombs CC, Roubinian JR, Talal N: Effect of androgen therapy on survival and suppressor activity in aged NZB/NZW F_1 hybrid mice. Clin Exp Immunol 52:229-233, 1983

18. Gershwin EM, Ahmed A, Steinberg AD, Thurman GB, Goldstein AL: Correction of T-cell function by thymosin in New Zealand mice. J Immunol 113:1068-1071, 1974

19. Seaman WE, Blackman MA, Greenspan JS, Talal N: Effect of ^{89}Sr on immunity and autoimmunity in NZB/NZW F_1 mice. J Immunol 124:812-818, 1980

20.   Fisher MS, Kripke ML: Systemic alteration induced in mice by ultraviolet light irradiation and its relationship to ultraviolet carcinogenesis. Proc Natl Acad Sci USA 74:1688-1692, 1977

21.   Noonan FP, DeFabo ED, Kripke ML: Suppression of contact hypersensitivity by UV irradiation and its relationship to UV-induced suppression of tumor immunity. Photochem Photobiol 34:683-689, 1981

22.   Letvin NL, Nepom JT, Greene MI, Benacerraf B, Germain RN: Loss of Ia-bearing splenic adherent cells after whole-body ultraviolet irradiation. J Immunol 125:2550-2554, 1980

ULTRAVIOLET-A1 (340-400 NM) IRRADIATION THERAPY IN SYSTEMIC LUPUS ERYTHEMATOSUS

H McGrath Jr[1], P Martinez-Osuna[1], FA Lee[2]

[1] Department of Medicine, Louisiana State University Medical Center, New Orleans; [2] Tulane/LSU General Clinical Research Center, Charity Hospital, New Orleans LA, USA

Source: Lupus 1996; 5, 269-274

Ultraviolet-A1 (UV-A1) wavelengths have been found effective in mitigating signs and symptoms of disease activity in systemic lupus erythematosus (SLE) but studies have been uncontrolled. To rigorously assess the effectiveness and safety of daily low-dose UV-A1 irradiation as a therapeutic agent in this disorder we enrolled 26 women with SLE in an 18-week two-phase study. During the initial six-week prospective, double-blind, placebo-controlled phase, the patients were divided into two groups; Group A was exposed to 60 kJ/m^2 of UV-A1 (340-400 nm) irradiation within a sunbed five days a week for three weeks and Group B was exposed for an equal amount of time to visible light of greater than > 430 nm (placebo). Each group was then crossed over for exposure to the other source for three weeks. During the second phase — 12 weeks — patients and physicians were unblinded and patients were irradiated with progressively decreasing levels of UV-A1 only.

Twenty-five patients completed the six-week placebo-controlled phase of the study and eighteen patients participated for the entire 18 weeks. In Group A the systemic lupus activity measure (SLAM) score improved significantly after three weeks of five-day-a-week UV-A1 irradiation ($P < 0.05$), regressing to baseline during the three weeks of placebo irradiation. Improvement recurred and progressed with six weeks of three-day-a-week UV-A1 irradiation ($P < 0.05$). Group B patients responded negligibly to the three weeks of visible light, more sharply to UV-A1, and as with Group A, maximally to the six weeks of three-day-a-week UV-A1 ($P < 0.01$). With twice- and then once-weekly UV-A1 irradiation the SLAM scores worsened slightly.

All patients decreased their drug use. Anti-double-stranded DNA antibodies (andi-dsDNA) decreased significantly ($P < 0.05$) and anti-nuclear antibodies non-significantly. Side effects were negligible. Visible light had no significant effect. In conclusion, low-dose UV-A1 irradiation effectively, comfortably, and without apparent toxicity diminished signs and symptoms of disease activity in SLE.

INTRODUCTION

Ultraviolet (UV) light sensitivity is characteristic of patients in SLE and UV-B (280-320 nm) wavelengths are the most toxic.[1] However, in animal studies exposure to wavelengths predominantly in the UV-A (320-400 nm) range had a paradoxically salutary effect on the disease, prolonging survival and decreasing anti-dsDNA levels and spleen size in the New Zealand Black/New Zealand White mouse model of SLE[2]. In an uncontrolled human study, irradiation with filtered TL/10R lamps emitting UV wavelengths exclusively in the UV-A1 (340-400 nm) range, significantly improved disease activity scores, decreasing rashes and photosensitivity, and in four of five patients decreasing or eliminating antibodies to SSA[3]. The present double-blind, placebo-controlled study was designed to test the effectiveness, safety and tolerance of low-dose UV-A1 radiation therapy in SLE.

PATIENTS AND METHODS

Twenty-six women with mild to moderate SLE, selected from private practices in the New Orleans area and from the Charity Hospital clinics in New Orleans, were included prospectively and allocated randomly to Group A (n = 14) or B (n = 12). Nineteen were white (nine in Group A, 10 in Group B), seven were black (five in Group A, two in Group B), and the mean age was 40.23 years (range 23-66 years, median 36 years). At entry, their disease had a mean duration of 8.56 years (range 0.8-27 years, median 5.5 years).

For inclusion, patients had to fulfill four or more American Rheumatism Association classification criteria for the diagnosis of SLE[4] and their disease had to be active as determined by the systemic lupus erythematosus activity measure (SLAM).[5] They were to make no change in their therapy for the two weeks prior to admission and no changes or additions (except for non-steroidal anti-inflammatory drugs and non-narcotic analgesics) throughout the initial six weeks, and after that only under our direction. Thirteen patients were taking prednisone (5-20 mg/day); five were taking hydroxychloroquine sulfate (200-400 mg/day); and all were using nonsteroidal anti-inflammatory drugs.

The initial placebo-controlled phase of the study lasted six weeks. Irradiation was carried out during the winter months to minimize concomitant exposure to natural sunlight. It consisted of 60kJ/m^2/day (about 0.15 of a minimal erythematous dose) of bodily UV-A1 irradiation five days a week for three weeks or an equivalent time exposure to visible light (placebo). Neither the examining physician nor the patient was aware of the irradiation source being used.

Patients in Group A were irradiated with UV-A1 for the first three weeks and then crossed over to placebo for three weeks. Conversely, patients in Group B were irradiated first with placebo for three weeks and then crossed over for three weeks of irradiation with UV-A1. Following this, all patients received only UV-A1 irradiation, 60 kJ/m^2 three times a week for six weeks, twice a week for three weeks, and then once a week for three weeks.

Irradiation was administered within bench-and-canopy type fan-cooled sunbeds (ALISUN '1000 combi', ALISUN Company, Eindhoven, The

Netherlands), and the patients wore undergarments and protective glasses. UV-A1 irradiation was delivered from TL/10R lamps (Philips International, Eindhoven, The Netherlands), 12 lamps in the canopy, protected by grids, and 12 in the bench, protected by a sheet of plexiglass 2028 that freely transmits all ultraviolet radiation. The grids and the plexiglass were covered with UVASUN-pink filters (MUTZHAS Co., Munich, Germany), 4 mm thick. Visible light was delivered from an identical arrangement but with the grids and plexiglass covered with UVASUN-yellow filters (MUTZHAS Co.). Midway through each treatment session, the patients were turned over once. UV-A1 irradiance at body surface was 87 W/m^2, and the duration of each irradiation was 11.5 min.

The irradiance of TL/10R lamps measured in one nm steps (data kindly supplied by BL Diffey, Durham, UL) has a spectrum of 340 nm to 450 nm, a peak wavelength of 365 nm with 99.01% UV-A1, 0.06% UV-B, 0.03% UV-A2 (320-340 nm) and 0% UV-C. The UVASUN-pink filters eliminate the UV-B and UV-A2 emission lines, transmitting ultraviolet radiation exclusively in the UV-A1 range. The UVASUN-yellow filters eliminate all wavelengths below 430 nm, transmitting only visible light. Ongoing UV-A1 measurements were made with an IL500 International Light Research Radiometer (International Light Inc., Newburyport, MA, USA), fitted with an SEE 015 photodiode and wide-eyed quartz diffuser covered by a UV-A filter measuring in the spectral range of 320-400 nm with peak response of 360 nm.

Disease activity was evaluated with the SLAM[5], filled out at baseline (average mean value of week —1 and week 1) and after 3, 6, 12, 15 and 18 weeks of therapy. This instrument lists 32 clinical and laboratory variables specific to the disease, each weighted from one to three according to their severity. The items are added and an aggregate score obtained. Two 100 mm visual analogue scales for measuring physician and patient global ratings from 'totally asymptomatic' to 'extremely symptomatic' accompany the SLAM.

On each patient a complete blood count (CBC), Westergren sedimentation rate (WSR) and urinalysis were done at the Charity Hospital Pathology Laboratories. The Tulane University Medical Center Immunology Laboratory determined antibody profiles using mouse kidney as substrate for the antinuclear antibody test (ANA) and

Ouchterlony double immunodiffusion on undiluted sera with commercially prepared antigens and house sera as controls for identifying antibodies to the antigens, Sjögren's syndrome A (SSA), Sjögren's syndrome B (SSB), ribonucleoprotein (RNP), Smith (Sm) and Scleroderma-70. They used a commercially available kit (Sanofi Diagnostics Pasteur, Inc., Chaska, MN, USA) with the *Crithidia lucilliae* kinetoplast as substrate for detective anti-dsDNA.

RESULTS

In Group A patients, the mean SLAM score decreased from a baseline of 8.4 ± 2.9 (n = 14) to 6.7 ± 1.9 (n = 13) ($P < 0.05$) after three weeks of five-day-a-week UV-A1 therapy, regressing after three weeks of placebo exposure to 8.5 ± 3.8 (n = 13). Improvement recurred and progressed with six weeks of three-day-a-week UV-A1 irradiation, the score dropping to 6.2 ± 3.3 (n = 9) ($P < 0.05$). In Group B patients, after three weeks of placebo irradiation, the SLAM score decreased marginally, from a baseline of 9.8 ± 4.2 to 9.7 ± 4.3 (n = 12) (P = NS), declining more sharply following three weeks of UV-A1 irradiation, to 8.4 ± 5.4 (n = 12) (P = NS), and decreasing further and significantly after six weeks of three-day-a-week UV-A1, to 5.3 ± 3.1 (n = 10) ($P < 0.01$). Thus, improvement peaked in both groups at week 12 after six weeks of three-times-a-week UV-A1 irradiation. Overall, further decreases in UV-A1 exposures to twice weekly and then once a week resulted in a partial loss of therapeutic effect, the score by week 18 increasing in Group A from 6.3 to 6.9 ± 4.3 (n = 8) (P = NS) and decreasing in Group B from 6.6 to 6.5 ± 2.8 (n = 9) (P = NS).

In seven of nine patients the ANA decrease by 1 titre in seven of 19 patients (P = NS) and the anti-dsDNA decreased by 1 or more titers in five of seven patients after three weeks of UV-A1 therapy ($P < 0.05$). Anti-Sm antibodies decreased in three of seven UV-A1-treated subjects after 18 weeks (P = NS). Lymphopenia resolved in two patients after 12 weeks and in one additional patient after 18 weeks of therapy (P = NS). The CBC, WSR, C3 and C4 did not change significantly. Placebo light had no significant effect on laboratory measures. As changes in laboratory measures were not pronounced, the changes in SLAM scores were governed predominantly by changes in clinical signs and symptoms of disease activity.

Twenty-five of the 26 patients enrolled completed the initial, six-week, double-blind phase of the study. During the extended 12 week phase, two patients were dropped for noncompliance, two because of slightly worsening discoid skin lesions and four because of lack of effect. The single patient who did not complete the initial phase was taking a photosensitizing drug and developed a transient rash. The response to UV-A1 irradiation took 7-10 days. Over half the patients detected minimal tanning after three weeks of UV-A1 exposure. At 12-15 weeks, the prednisone dosage could be tapered by at least 50% in two and discontinued in three of 13 patients; all decreased non-steroidal anti-inflammatory drug use; hydroxychloroquine sulfate dosages were unchanged. By 18 weeks, 13 of the 17 patients reported a lower frequency of flares. All but one of the patients completing the 18 weeks chose to continue treatment beyond the scope of this study because of the benefits experienced.

DISCUSSION

Low-dose UV-A1 irradiation mitigated signs and symptoms of disease activity in patients with SLE, with optimal therapeutic action occurring after the administration of 60 kJ/m^2 three times a week. The effect was demonstrated best among those patients treated first with three weeks of UV-A1 irradiation; they improved significantly during the UV-A1 irradiation, regressed to baseline during visible light irradiation and then again responded to UV-A1, this time maximally, despite fewer weekly doses of irradiation. The patients who were started on placebo showed essentially no response to placebo but a good response to UV-A1 irradiation, again maximally and significantly after the six-week, three-day-a-week exposure. Although the therapy attenuated constitutional and other symptoms, there is no evidence that it eliminates the underlying disease or the need for continued close monitoring by a physician. Long-term follow-up studies indicate that patients maintain their improved status with two- or three-times-a-week irradiations of 80-100 kJ/m^2, but that decreases in this level invariably bring recrudescence of symptoms (manuscript in preparation).

The remedial action of low-dose UV-A1 irradiation seems at variance with the established toxicity of UV-B irradiation in SLE.[1] However, it should be appreciated that there is a discordance and often an antagonism between the actions of these two wavelength bands, those of UV-A1 often countering the disease-based aberrancies in SLE, while those of UV-B promote them. For example, UV-B wavelengths are readily absorbed by DNA[6], a major autoantigen in SLE. The resulting generation of cyclobutane thymine dimers enhances DNA immunogenicity[7]. DNA, altered or unaltered[8], is released into the circulation[9], where it can bind with pre-formed anti-DNA antibodies. On the contrary, UV-A1 photons, weakly absorbed by and therefore not directly damaging to DNA[10], promote photo-reactivation[11], a process directed at the repair of DNA cyclobutane pyrimidine dimers whether these are UV-B induced or secondary to other insults.

Additionally, UV-B radiation downregulates antigen presenting function, inducing CD1a- DR+ antigen presenting cells[12], cis urocanic acid[13] and epidermal suppressor factor[14], all of which suppress cell-mediated immunity (CMI), which is already impaired in SLE[15]. On the other hand, UV-A1 photons enhance CMI, presumably by failing to generate CD1a-DR+ antigen-presenting cells within the epidermis and by enhancing the production of CD1a+ DR+ cells[16] that promote CMI[12]. UV-A1 radiation also generates the production of *cis*-urocanic acid and an epidermal suppressor factor that fail to suppress CMI *in vivo*[13,14], apparently, at least in the case of urocanic acid, because UV-A1 is inhibiting the immunosuppression[13]. The resistance to and sometimes exacerbation by UV-A1 radiation of discoid LE lesions observed in the present study is consistent with a promotion of CMI by UV-A1, since discoid LE has a T cell-mediated immune basis[17].

The reciprocal propensities of UV-B and UV-A1 radiation also may play a role in the recently described propensity for UV-B but not UV-A1 photons to promote translocation of soluble non-histone nuclear antigens to the surface of cells[18]. This translocation phenomenon, upregulated in SLE patients[19], triggers cell lysis through antibody-mediated cytotoxicity in those SLE patients who possess antibodies to the intra-cellular antigens. The effectiveness of UV-A1 photons in ameliorating rashes in particular subacute cutaneous lupus erythematosus (SCLE)[4], an SLE variant linked to the translocation phenomenon[20], suggests an inhibitory role for UV-A1 photons.

A unique action of UV-A1 photons that has remedial potential is their capacity to induce immediate apoptosis[21]. A form of programmed cell death directed at eliminating cells that are no longer necessary for, or that may interfere with normal human development, apoptosis is thought to be defective, blocked or inhibited in SLE[22]. Although all UV wavelengths induce delayed transcriptional apoptosis, only those of UV-A1, through the generation of reactive oxygen species, bring about immediate non-transcriptional apoptosis[21]. Acting in a supplemental or preemptive mode, this relatively clean and noninflammatory type of programmed cell death would seem preferable in SLE to the alternatives[23]: liquefaction degeneration or necrosis with spillover of phlogistic cellular constituents into the circulation, or non-death leading to persistence and proliferation of activated autoimmune lymphocytes.

Whether through immediate apoptosis, DNA repair or enhancement of CMI, it seems inescapable that the skin and in particular the dermal-epidermal (D-E) junction, as primary targets of UV-A1 photon bombardment, are major transducers of its beneficial actions. In our view, dampening disease activity within the D-E junction, perhaps the most consistently autoreactive and chronically simmering inflammatory site of involvement in SLE[24], reduces not only dermal manifestations of disease but also the joint pain and constitutional symptoms that result from spillover of D-E constituents into the circulation.

The deeply penetrating UV-A1 photons[25] may also effect a systemic 'reach' through their direct impact on peripheral mononuclear cells that circulate and percolate through the epidermis or by modulating the release of soluble mediators from UV-A1 irradiated skin. UV-A1 wavelengths do not elicit their action via the optic-pineal-hypothalamic pathway as the patients' eyes are covered during therapy.

In sharp contrast to the observed benefits of UV-A1 radiation are recent reports of UV-A and even UV-A1 radiation toxicity in SLE patients with exposure to these wavelengths inducing earlier and more persistent erythema and sometimes eliciting rashes in SLE patients compared with normals. However, the wavelengths used differed from our own; for example one group of investigators[26] irradiated patients with levels of UV-A an order of magnitude higher than ours and inclusive of UV-A2 (320-340 nm), a band of wavelengths now considered to be functionally an extension of UV-B[27]. A case of report of phototoxicity due to UV-A emissions from a photocopier machine[28] can be explained similarly. In a third study, investigators[29] employed monochromatic wavelengths that were approximately 2 orders of magnitude greater in intensity than any individual wavelength within our polychromatic UV-A1 spectrum; in a fourth study, investigators found UV-A wavelengths to be without toxicity.[30]

Of the two patients who dropped out of our study because of a diffuse rash, one experienced considerable symptomatic relief but was taking a photosensitizer, diltiazem, that induced sunburn and could not be replaced because of the patient's drug allergies. The other patient insisted, contrary to our observations, that she noted a rash; she had receved only 10 days of placebo light.

Since the therapy is long term, it should be noted that 38 of 47 albino hairless mice, highly susceptible to skin tumors, developed 1 mm tumors after a median of 265 days of daily exposure to 220 kJ/m^2 of UV-A1 radiation[31]. There has been no reported incidence of skin tumors in humans treated with high dose (1300 kJ/m^2) UV-A1 radiation for atopic dermatitis.[16]

In conclusion, UV-A1 photons delivered dermally at low levels at patients with SLE, effectively, comfortably and progressively relieved constitutional and other signs and symptoms of disease activity; reduced the need for medication; and attenuated autoimmune antibody levels. We propose that these deeply penetrating photons implement their benefits primarily by quelling simmering inflammation within the skin, a massive organ that can contribute considerable phlogistic overflow in SLE. The effectiveness of UV-A1 radiation therapy is provocative, offering both a new avenue of SLE therapy and a new perspective on the complex role ultraviolet light in this disorder.

ACKNOWLEDGEMENTS

We are indebted to Ms Julie Basco and Ms Sandra Toups for assistance in preparing the manuscript, Dr Peter Kohler and the staff at Tulane/LSU General Clinical Research Center for their cooperation and support, and to Anne Compliment and Azzudin E Gharavi, MD for their assistance in editing the manuscript. Supported by the National Institutes of Health grant RRO5096-06, Tulane/LSU General Clinical Research Center, Charity Hospital, New Orleans, LA, USA and the Louisiana Lupus Foundation, Baton Rouge, LA, USA.

REFERENCES

1. Cripps DJ, Rankin J. Action spectra of lupus erythematosus and experimental immunofluorescence. *Arch Dermatol* 1973; **107**; 563-567.

2. McGrath H Jr, Bak E, Michalski JP. Ultraviolet-A light prolongs survival and improves immune function in (New Zealand black X New Zealand white) F_1 hybrid mice. *Arthritis Rheum* 1987; **30**; 557-561.

3. McGrath H. Ultraviolet-A1 irradiation decreases clinical disease activity and autoantibodies in patients with systemic lupus erythematosus. *Clin Exp Rheum* 1994; **12**; 129-135.

4. Tan EM *et al.* The 1982 revised criteria for the classification of systemic lupus erythematosus. *Arthritis Rheum* 1982; **25**; 1271-1277.

5. Liang MH, Socher SA, Larson MG, Schur PH. Reliability and validity of six systems for the clinical assessment of disease activity in systemic lupus erythematosus. *Arthritis Rheum* 1989; **32**; 1107-1118.

6. Setlow RB. Wavelengths in sunlight effective in producing skin cancer. A theoretical analysis. *Proc Natl Acad Sci* 1974; USA **71**; 3363-3366.

7. Davis P, Russel AS, Percy JS. Antibodies to UV light denatured DNA in systemic lupus erythematosus. *J Rheumatol* 1976; **3**; 375-379.

8. Tan EM. In: Miescher RA (ed) *Immunopathology: Sixth international symposium* Basil:Schwabe, 1971, 36-38.

9. Golan D, Borel Y. Spontaneous increase of DNA turnover in murine systemic lupus erythematosus. *E J Immunol* 1983; **13**; 430-433.

10. Sutherland JC, Griffen KP. Absorption spectrum of DNA for wavelengths longer than 320 nm. *Radiat Res* 1981; **86**; 399-409.

11. Sutherland BM, Hacham H, Grange RW, Sutherland JC. Pyrimidine dimer formation by UVA radiation: implications for

photo-reactivation. In: Urbach FA (ed) *Biologic responses to UVA irradiation.* Valdenmar: Kansas City, 1991, 47-58.

12. Baadsgaard O, MD, Wulf HC, Wantzin GL, Cooper KD, UVB and UVC, but not UVA, potently induce the appearance of T6-DR+ antigen-presenting cells in human epidermis. *J Invest Dermatol* 1987; **89**; 113-118.

13. DeFabo EC, Reilly DC, Noonan FP: Mechanism of UVA effects on immune function: preliminary studies. In: Urbach FA, (ed) *Biologic responses to UVA radiation.* Valdenmar: Kansas City, 1991, 227-237.

14. Kim TY, Kripke ML, Ullrich SE. Immunosuppression by factors released from UV-irradiated epidermal cells: selective effects on the generation of contact and delayed hypersensitivities after exposure to UVA or UVB radiation. *J Invest Dermatol* 1990; **94**; 26-32.

15. Horowitz DA. Impaired delayed type hypersensitivity in systemic lupus erythematosus. *Arthritis Rheum* 1972; **15**; 353-359.

16. Krutmann J *et al.* High dose UVA1 therapy in the treatment of patients with atopic dermatitis. *J Am Acad Dermatol* 1992; **26**; 225-230.

17. Synkowski DR, Provost TT. Characterization of the inflammation in lupus erythematosus lesions using monoclonal antibodies. *J Rheumatol* 1983; **10**; 920-924.

18. Furukawa F, Kanauchi H, Imamura S. Susceptibility to UVB light in cultured keratinocytes of cutaneous lupus erythematosus. *Dermatology* 1994; **189S:1**; 18-23.

19. Golan TD, Elkon KB, Gharavi AE, Krueger JG. Enhanced membrane binding of autoantibodies to cultured keratinocytes of systemic lupus erythematosus patients after ultraviolet A/B irradiation. *J Clin Invest* 1992; **90**; 1067-1072.

20. Sontheimer RD, McCauliffe DP. Pathogenesis of anti-Ro/SS-A autoantibody-associated cutaneous lupus erythematosus. *Dermatol Clin* 1990; **8**; 751-758.

21. Godar DE, Lucas AD. Spectral dependence of UV-induced immediate and delayed apoptosis: the role or membrane and DNA damage. *Photochem Photobiol* 1995; **62**; 108-113.

22. Carron DA, Tan EM. Apoptosis in rheumatic disease. *Bull Rheum Dis* 1995; **44**; 1-3.

23. Searle J, Kerr JFR, Bishop CJ. Necrosis and apoptosis: distinct modes of cell death with fundamentally different significance. *Pathol Annu* 1982; **17(pt 2)**; 229-259.

24. Tuffanelli DL, Kay D, Fukuyama K. Dermal-epidermal junction in lupus erythematosus. *Arch Dermatol* 1969; **99**; 652-662.

25. Bruls WAG, Slaper H, Van Der Leun JC, Berrens L. Transmission of human epidermis and stratum corneum as a function of thickness in the ultraviolet and visible wavelengths. *Photochem Photobiol* 1984; **40**; 485-494.

26. Lehrmann P *et al.* Experimental reproduction of skin lesions in lupus erythematosus by UVA and UVB radiation. *J Am Acad Dermatol* 1989; **22**; 181-187.

27. Kochevar IE. Acute effects of ultraviolet radiation on skin. In: Holick MF, Kligman AM (eds) *Biologic effects of light.* Walter DeGruyter: New York, 1992, 1-10.

28. Klein LR, Elmets CA, Callen JP. Photoexacerbation of cutaneous lupus erythematosus due to ultraviolet A emissions from a photocopier. *Arthritis Rheum* 1995; **38**; 1152-1156.

29. Nived O, Johansen PB, Sturfeld G. Standardized ultraviolet-A exposure provokes skin reaction in systemic lupus erythematosus. *Lupus* 1993; **2**; 247-250.

30. Wolska H, Blaszczyk M, Jablonska S. Phototests in patients with various forms of lupus erythematosus. *Int J Dermatol* 1989; 98-102.

31. Sterenborg H, van der Leun J. Tumorigenesis by a long wavelength UV-A Source. *Photochem Photobiol* 1990; 325-330.

LONGTERM ULTRAVIOLET-A1 IRRADIATION THERAPY IN SLE

JOSE F. MOLINA, MD, Rheumatology Fellow and HUGH McGRATH Jr, MD, Professor of Medicine, Sectionof Rheumatology, Louisiana State University Medical Center, New Orleans, USA

Original, unedited source:
The Journal of Rheumatology 1997; 24:1072-1074

ABSTRACT

Objective: In a recent series of short term research studies ultraviolet-A1 (UVA1; 340-400 nm) dermal irradiation proved effective in reducing the signs and symptoms of SLE disease activity in patients. To determine if this positive effect persists with longer term therapy, we followed the progress of 6 patients for an average of 3.4 years (range 2.4-4.5 years). The 6 subjects had significant decreases in signs and symptoms of disease activity during the first 12 weeks of the earlier studies while receiving 3 to 5 low dose UVA1 irradiations weekly and were asked to continue therapy.

Methods: Long term therapy consisted of 1 or 2 irradiations of 6-15 J/m^2 (15-30 minutes, or about 1/8-1/4 of the Minimal Erythema Dose) each week. We assessed patient progress every 3 months with systemic lupus activity measures.

Results: Despite the smaller number of weekly treatments, the gains achieved during the initial 12 weeks of UVA1 therapy, not only continued but slightly increased. Skin tanning was moderate to absent, the therapy was tolerated well, and there was no noted toxicity.

Conclusion: UVA1 radiation induced remissions in SLE patients persist with longer term therapy; 1 or 2 weekly exposures suffice; there appears to be no toxicity of significance.

Although the shortest wavelength band of terrestrial ultraviolet radiation, known as UVB (280-320 nm) is well established to be toxic to SLE[1] patients, we have observed that exposure to the longer wavelength bands — UVA (320-400 nm) in animals[2] and UVA1 (340-400 nm) in humans[3,4,5] — is therapeutic in this disease. In uncontrolled studies[3,4] and more recently, in a 26 patient, 12 week prospective, double blind, placebo controlled crossover trial[5], UVA1 (340-400 nm) radiation exposures significantly decreased the symptoms of SLE disease activity. We describe the progress of 6 SLE patients from earlier studies who agreed to enter long term treatment.

MATERIALS AND METHODS

Six SLE patients from earlier studies who had met the American College of Rheumatology (ACR) criteria for SLE[6] entered the long term study. Along with most other patients they had experienced significant decreases in the symptoms of SLE disease activity during the first 12 weeks of the earlier studies while receiving 3 to 5 low dose UVA1 irradiations each week. In this long term study, their UVA1 (340-400 nm) dermal irradiation therapy consisted of 1 or 2 irradiations of 6-15 J/m^2 (15-30 min or about 1/8-1/4 of the minimal erythema dose) per week. Due to unavoidable scheduling circumstances, on occasion 1 or 2 week lapses in therapy occurred early in this procedure. Patient progress was assessed with the systemic lupus activity measures (SLAM)[7] established at baseline, 12 weeks, and every 3 months thereafter. SLAM lists 25 clinical and 7 laboratory variables specific to SLE, each weighted 0 to 3 according to severity. The clinical variables fall under 10 major headings: constitutional, integument, eye, reticuloendothelial, pulmonary, cardiovascular, gastrointestinal, neuromotor, joints, and other. The 7 laboratory variables are complete blood count (CBC), serum creatinine, and urine sediment (Westergren ESR). The 32 items are then added together to obtain an aggregate score. Two 100 mm visual analog scales for measuring both physician and patient ratings from "totally asymptomatic" to "extremely symptomatic" accompany the SLAM.

The irradiation methodology has been previously described[4,5]. UVA1 irradiation is delivered by Philips TL/10R lamps covered with a UVA-SUN Mutzhas filter. The patient lies in a fan-cooled, 24-lamp sunbed and turns over once midway through the treatment session. The UV irradiance emitted is 100 percent UVA1 (340-400 nm) and the irradiance incident on the body's surface is 87 W/m^2.

The irradiance of TL/10R lamps measured in one nm steps has a spectrum of 340 to 450 nm, a peak wavelength of 365 nm, with 99.01 percent UVA1 (340-400 nm), 0.065 percent UVB (280-320 nm), 0.035 percent UVA2 (320-340 nm), and 0 percent UVC (100-280 nm). The

UVASUN filters totally eliminate all of the UVB and UVA2 wavelengths, transmitting UVA1 radiation exclusively.

Statistical analysis. Descriptive statistics were performed and the differences between means and proportions were established using one way analysis of variance (ANOVA) and a nonparametric test (Tukey-Kramer multiple comparisons test). A p value of < 0.05 was designated to be statistically significant.

RESULTS

All of the patients who improved significantly in the earlier studies kept, and even slightly increased, this improvement during the long term study (average 3.4 years). The mean SLAM score, which had decreased from a baseline of 14 ± 4.8 to 7.6 ± 3.5 after the first 12 weeks of treatments (p < 0.05) during the earlier studies, decreased even further to 6.4 ± 2.3 after 3.4 years (p < 0.01). The CBC, ESR, C3, C4, urinalysis, and chemistry 12 screen, which did not significantly change in the earlier studies, did not change during this long term followup study either. The antinuclear and anti-SSA antibodies that had become negative in earlier studies in Patients #6 and #1, remained negative during the long term study. Although patient drug needs had decreased in earlier studies, the drugs and their doses remained basically unchanged during the long term research study.

All patients complained of disease exacerbations, mainly fatigue and joint pain, during unscheduled 1 or 2 week lapses early in the therapy. Because these lapses were unplanned they were not monitored with SLAM measures. Skin tanning was negligible to modest, treatments were tolerated well, and there was no observed toxicity.

Oral ulcers, rashes, joint pain, photosensitivity, sleeping patterns, and headaches which were responsive in the short term studies continued to positively respond during this longer term trial. However, no other single response was more gratifying to the patients than the sustained relief of their fatigue. Patients reported either returning to work or increasing their workloads, and made known a marked improvement in the overall quality of their lives because of their new found energy.

DISCUSSION

This study supports several observations made during the short term investigations. First of all, the sometimes striking reduction of rashes, joint pain, and other constitutional symptoms that were seen during the short term studies continued, and even diminished further. Second, although we had conducted therapy with 3 to 5 weekly treatments in the first studies, an average of 2 irradiations per week proved sufficient in this study. With less than 2 weekly irradiations, patients reported an increase in symptoms, so that very early in the study they became resolute about coming regularly for treatments, despite any inconvenience that might cause. Third, the treatments continued to be without any apparent toxicity.

Although the mechanisms underlying this salutary action are unknown, it is reasonable to assume that either much or most of the ameliorative action of UVA1 is mediated through the skin, the body's largest organ. Characterized by widespread heightened immunoreactivity within the dermal-epidermal junction[8,9], the skin of SLE patients has the potential to contribute to the circulation a large overflow of inflammatory constituents capable of increasing the systemic manifestations of disease activity. UVA1 photons appear able to attenuate this dermal immunoreactive/inflammatory aberration. There is some evidence they enhance T cell mediated immunity[10,11], suppressed in SLE[12], and suppress humoral immunity[13], enhanced in SLE. Through a process of photoreactivation they also repair damaged DNA[14], immunogenic in SLE[15]. They decrease serum levels of interleukin 12 (unpublished observation), plentiful in keratinocytes and a mediator of both antibody dependent cellular cytotoxicity and T cell cytotoxicty[16,17], mechanisms described as underlying the keratinocyte lysis responsible for the dermal inflammatory responses in both SLE[18] and subactue cutaneous lupus.

Although it might be possible the deep penetrating UVA1 photons may also have a more direct systemic reach through their penetration to the mononuclear cells which are circulating through the epidermis[19,20], the short duration of UVA1 exposures during treatment sessions seems too brief for any substantial effect.

Observations of both short and long term effects of UVA1 therapy for SLE are consistent with other findings over the past 15 years, namely, that the photobiological properties of UV wavelengths above and below 340 nm differ markedly[21] from one another. We found disease activity in SLE, though exacerbated by short UV wavelengths, was attenuated by the longer UVA1 wavelengths. Long term, low dose UVA1 therapy maintained the gains made during the shorter term therapy, with 1 to 3 weekly exposures being sufficient for this continuity. The UVA1 light therapy was well tolerated, without any apparent toxicity, and is easily administered to patients. Its effectiveness not only suggests a new manner of therapy for the SLE patient, but it also offers a new perspective on the complex role UV light plays in lupus.

REFERENCES

1.   Cripps DJ, Rankin J: Action spectra of lupus erythematosus and experimental immunofluorescence. *Arch Dermatol 1973*; 107:563-7.

2.   McGrath H Jr, Bak E, Michalski JP: Ultraviolet-A light prolongs survival and improves immune function in (New Zealand black x New Zealand white)F_1 hybrid mice. *Arthritis Rheum 1987*; 30:557-61.

3.   McGrath H Jr, Bell JM, Haynes MR, Martinez-Osuna P: Ultraviolet-A irradiation therapy for patients with systemic lupus erythematosus: A pilot study. *Curr Ther Res 1994*; 55:373-81.

4.   McGrath H: Ultraviolet-A1 irradiation decreases clinical disease activity and autoantibodies in patients with systemic lupus erythematosus. *Clin Exp Rheumatol 1994*; 12:129-35.

5.   Martinez O, Suna P, McGrath H Jr, Lee FA: Ultraviolet-A1 (340-400 nm) irradiation therapy in systemic lupus erythematosus. *Lupus 1996*; 5:269-74.

6.   Tan EM, Cohen AS, Fries JF, *et al*: The 1982 revised criteria for classification of systemic lupus erythematosus. *Arthritis Rheum 1982*; 25:1271-7.

7.   Liang MH, Socher SA, Larson MG, Schur PH: Reliability and validity of six systems for the clinical assessment of disease

activity in systemic lupus erythematosus. *Arthritis Rheum 1989*; 32:1107-18.

8.   Tuffanelli D, Kay D, Fukuyama K: Dermal-epidermal junction in lupus erythematosus. *Arch Dermatol 1969*; 99:652-62.

9.   Provost TT, Guiseppe A, Maddison PJ, Reichlin M: Lupus band test in untreated SLE patients: Correlation of immunoglobulin deposition in the skin of the extensor forearm with clinical renal disease and serological abnormalities. *J Invest Dermatol 1980*; 74:407-12.

10.   Morison WL, Pike RA, Kripke ML: Effect of sunlight and its component wavebands on contact hypersensitivity in mice and guinea pigs. *Photodermatology 1985*; 2:195-204.

11.   Hager ED, Benninghoff BB, Pakdaman A, Stickl A, Mutzhas MF: Vergesserung zellvermittelter Immunitat bei Tumorpatienten durch hochdosierte Phototherapie mit lan-welligem Ultraviolett-A (UV-A1). *Deutsche Zeitschrift fur Onkologie 1989*; 2:42-9.

12.   Horowitz DA: Impaired delayed type hypersensitivity in systemic lupus erythematosus. *Arthritis Rheum 1972*; 15:353-9.

13.   Godar DE, Beer JZ: UVA1-induced anuclear damage in mammalian cells. In: Urbach FA, ed. *Biological Responses to UVA Irradiation*. Kansas City: Valdenmar, 1991:65-73.

14.   Sutherland BM, Hacham H, Grange RW, Sutherland JC: Pyrimidine dimer formation by UVA radiation: Implications for photoreactivation. In: Urbach FA, ed. *Biological Responses to UVA Irradiation*. Kansas City: Valdenmar, 1991:47-58.

15.   Tan EM, Stoughton RB: Ultraviolet light alteration of cellular deoxyribonucleic acid *in vivo*. *Proc Natl Acad Sci 1969*; 62:708-14.

16.   Lieberman MD, Sigal RK, Williams NN, Daly JM: Natural killer cell stimulatory factor augments natural killer cell and antibody-dependent tumoricidal response against colon carcinoma cell lines. *J Surg Res 1991*; 50:410-5.

17.   Trinchieri G: Interleukin-12: A cytokine produced by antigen presenting cells with immunoregulatory functions in the generation of T-helper cells type 1 and cytotoxic lymphocytes. *Blood 1994*; 84:4008-27.

18.   Norris DA, Ryan SR, Fritz KA, *et al:* The role of RNP, Sm and SS-A/Ro-specific antisera from patients with lupus erythematosus in inducing antibody-dependent cellular cytotoxicity of targets coated with nonhistone nuclear antigens. *Clin Immunol Immunopathol 1984*; 31:311-20.

19.   Bruls WAG, Slaper H, Van Der Leun JC, Berrens L: Transmission of human epidermis and stratum corneum as a function of thickness in the ultraviolet and visible wavelengths. *Photochem Photobiol 1984*; 40:485-94.

20.   McGrath H Jr, Wilson WA, Scopelitis E: Acute effects of low-fluence ultraviolet light on human T-lymphocyte subsets. *Photochem Photobiol 1986*; 627-31.

21.   Kochevar IE: Acute effects of ultraviolet radiation on skin. In: Holick, MF, Kligman AM, eds. *Biologic Effects of Light*. New York: Walter DeGruyter, 1992:1-10.

PROSPECTS FOR UV-A1 THERAPY AS A TREATMENT MODALITY IN CUTANEOUS AND SYSTEMIC LE

H. MCGRATH Jr.

Department of Medicine, Section of Rheumatology, Louisiana State University Medical School, 1542 Tulane Ave., New Orleans, LA 70112 and The Tulane/LSU General Clinic Research Center, Charity Hospital, New Orleans, LA 70112, USA

Source: Lupus 1997; 6, 209-217

INTRODUCTION

The noxious effects of UV radiation in SLE are well known.[1,2] However, patients and physicians have long appreciated that the longer UV wavelengths designated as ultraviolet-A (UV-A: 320-400nm) lack the toxicity of the shorter UV wavelengths known as ultraviolet-B (UV-B: 280-320nm).[1,2] Additionally, some years ago evidence began to appear in the literature that UV-A and UV-B wavelengths have dissociated[3,4] or even opposing[5,6] actions along the immunological and photochemical lines, raising the possibility that some long UV lengths have beneficial effects in SLE.

Testing the action of UV-A1 radiation is an animal model of lupus

We tested the action of UV-A irradiation in the New Zealand Black/New Zealand White F1 hybrid (B/W) mouse model of lupus.[7] Over a seven month period, we observed that B/W mice irradiated with low-dose UV-A survived at a time when 60% of the non-irradiated controls died along a mortality curve standard for this strain.[8] Sacrifice of the surviving mice revealed that the irradiated mice had significantly smaller spleens ($P < 0.05$), lower anti-double-stranded DNA antibody (anti-ds DNA) ($P < 0.05$), and more normal splenic lymphocyte function ($P < 0.01$) than did the non-irradiated mice. Exposure to UV-A wavelengths appeared to be note only harmless but remedial.

UV-A1 radiation in humans with SLE

We proceeded cautiously to study UV-A irradiation in humans with SLE. However, because the 'black lamps' used as our source of UV-A radiation in the mouse study emitted moderate amounts of UV-B wavelengths, toxic in SLE, this source was unacceptable for our human studies. Even the shorter UV-A wavelengths — from 320-340 nm (UV-A2) were considered undesirable because investigators were increasingly aware that their properties overlapped those of UV-B.[9] We searched for a UV-A source lacking these shorter UV wavelengths and secured from the Philips Company (Eindhoven, The Netherlands) the TL/10R lamp that generates UV radiation, 99.1% of which is UV-A1 (340-400 nm), 0.06% UV-B, and 0.03% UV-A2.

In an open clinical trial, we irradiated 15 patients within a sunbed with 65 kJ/m^2/d of radiation from TL/10R lamps five days a week for three weeks.[10] This low-dose treatment brought about significant decreases in fatigue, joint pain, fever, malaise, and morning-stiffness ($P < 0.05$), and in physician/patient assessment of disease activity ($P < 0.01$). Overall clinical disease activity ($P < 0.01$) decreased from a score of 15.4±1.5-10±0.01. White blood cell and platelet counts increased ($P < 0.05$), percentages of CD4, 4B4, and 2H4 cells decreased ($P < 0.05$), and B-cell percentages decreased by 18% ($P < 0.07$).

We were encouraged by these results and by the paucity of short UV wavelengths emitted from our irradiation source, a welcome safety factor. Nevertheless, because of the established toxicity of these shorter UV wavelengths in SLE and the evidence from out study and others[11] that even these low levels of short-wavelength UV radiation were photoimmunologically active, namely, reducing lymphocyte counts and CD4/CD8 in humans, we opted to eliminate all UV-B and UV-A2 radiation in the belief that it might be undermining the benefits of UV-A1 radiation in SLE.

Eliminating all UV wavelengths less than 340 nm from the irradiation source

In our second open trial, we covered the TL/10R lamps with UVASUN-pink filters (Mutzhas Co., Munich, Germany) that absorb all UV wavelengths below 340nm, allowing emission of only UV-A1 wavelengths. Ten SLE patients were irradiated for 15 d, four of them for eight months, with 60 kJ/m^2/d of UV-A1 irradiation, approximately 1/6-1/8 of the dose needed to produce minimal erythema in the average Caucasian. Significant decreases in clinical disease activity resulted, greater than those in the first study.[12] Moreover, although clinical indices of the 10 patients had decreased by 30% after three weeks, the improvement in the four patients irradiated for eight months decreased by 70%. Surprisingly, the 5 SSA patients had a decrease or disappearance of antibodies to SSA. Among these five several experienced abatement of their severe photosensitivity and one had striking resolution of a severe, long-standing, corticosteroid-resistant, diffuse, beefy erythematous rash of subacute cutaneous lupus erythematosus (SCLE). The results indicated that pure UV-A1 irradiation had the potential to decrease clinical signs and symptoms of disease and decrease SSA antibody titers and that these effects persisted or increased with time.

Not long after this, another patient with SCLE severe enough, along with her associated arthritis and fatigue, to keep her housebound and virtually bed-ridden for four years, responded strikingly to UV-A1 therapy. Prednisone and hydroxychloroquine had long been ineffective in resolving her disease manifestations but daily UV-A1 exposures completely resolved her severe dermatitis within three weeks, while relieving her constitutional symptoms. Before and after photographs attest to the dermal response. Less frequent exposures have maintained her, resulting in her entering fully again into the mainstream of activities in her household and community.

The effectiveness of UV-A1 photons in ameliorating photosensitivity and SCLE rashes[12,13] — both commonly associated with SSA antibody — and the observed decreases in SSA antibody levels with this treatment, raise the prospect of preventing or ameliorating other SSA antibody-associated syndromes, such as neonatal lupus[14] — with or without complete heart block — of SSA unclassified connective tissue disease[15], with this therapy.

Possible mechanisms of UV-A1 radiation action in SLE

The remedial action of low-dose UV-A1 irradiation seems at variance with the established toxicity of UV-B irradiation in SLE. Nevertheless, our preliminary observations that the longer UV wavelengths had healing properties held promise not only as a new avenue of therapy but as a means of securing critical insights into the forces that drive disease activity in SLE. Why would it work?

Falling within the electromagnetic spectrum between X-rays and visible light, UV radiation has conventionally been divided into wavelength bands of increasing length and decreasing energy and toxicity. Vacuum UV (< 200 nm), UV-C (200-260 nm), UV-B, and UV-A encompass the spectrum, with UV-B and UV-A being the only terrestrial wavelengths. In recent years a further demarcation has become necessary; because they appear to be in a class of their own, wavelengths between 340-400 nm have been designated UV-A1, and those wavelengths from 320-340 nm, UV-A2.[9] The properties of the UV-A2 band increasingly appear to be an extension of UV-B[9] and the actions of UV-A1 wavelengths as dissociated from or antagonistic to those of the shorter wavelengths.[16,17,18] In fact, UV-A1 radiation may be more closely related to visible light[19] than to the shorter UV wavelengths. A major — perhaps the major — spectral break within the range of terrestrial ultraviolet wavelengths is fast becoming recognized as approximately 340 nm.

UV-A1 action transmitted through the skin

Inasmuch as the primary target of UV-A1 radiation is the skin, it is reasonable to conclude that the action of its photons is transduced through this massive organ. Due to the propensities of UV-A1 photons to promote DNA repair,[5,16] enhance cell-mediated immunity,[18] trigger immediate apoptosis,[20] alter Th1/Th2 profiles,[21] and possibly interfere with translocation,[22,23] this band of wavelengths is well poised to play a remedial role in SLE, in marked contrast to the actions of UV-B photons, which exacerbate disease. The direct dampening of disease activity within the dermal-epidermal (D-E) junctions — perhaps the most consistently autoreactive and chronically simmering inflammatory site of involvement in SLE[24] — should itself suffice to reduce not only the dermal manifestations of disease but the joint pain and constitutional symptoms that result from spillover of phlogistic constituents from the D-E junction into the circulation. In order to understand the beneficial potential of UV-A1 photons, it's helpful to contrast their action with those of UV-B, which are toxic in SLE.

To begin with, UV-B radiation is absorbed strongly by DNA,[25] a major autoantigen in SLE.[26] DNA damage results, manifesting as DNA photoproducts, the most plentiful of which are the immunogenic cyclobutane pyrimidine dimers.[27] The release of both dimers and unaltered DNA into the circulation[28,29] results in the enhancement of DNA immunogenicity[30] and to the binding of DNA by pre-formed anti-dsDNA, leading to immune complex-induced tissue damage. In contrast, UV-A1 photons pass relatively freely through DNA,[3] doing no damage. Indeed, through a process known as photoreactivation, UV-A1 photons and the shorter visible wavelengths promote repair of damaged DNA in animals.[5,16]

The action of the different wavelengths on cell-mediated immunity, which is depressed in SLE,[31] is equally germane to an understanding of UV-A1 benefits. As highly effective suppressors of CMI,[32] UV-B wavelengths represent potentiators of this deficit in SLE. UV-A1, as an enhancer of CMI,[7,18] has a beneficial portent. Unlike UV-B photons, which promote enrichment of the epidermis with CD — DR + cells, which are suppressors of CMI,[33] UV-A1 photons generate a predominance of CD + DR + cells, upregulators of CMI.[17] UV-B wavelengths generate cis-urocanic acid[34] and epidermal suppressor factor,[35] which suppress CMI, whereas UV-A1 radiation generates these same mediators devoid of suppressor activity.[34,35] Our observations of non-responsiveness and, occasionally, a slight worsening of discoid lesions after UV-A1 radiation, despite the striking responsiveness of SCLE rashes,[12] is consistent with UV-A1-induced enhancement of CMI. Discoid lupus is a T-cell-mediated disorder,[36] while SCLE has the earmarks of an antibody-mediated disorder; it is ANA-dependent,[37] characterized by the presence of intradermal IgG deposits[38] and a D-E junctional membrane attack complex,[39] and evinces evidence of antibody-dependence cell cytotoxicity (ADCC) mediated damage.[40]

In humans with SLE UV-B photons suppress[32,33] an already impaired [31,41] T-cell-mediated immunity while sparing humoral immune responsiveness,[42] effectively decreasing Th1/Th2 cytokine profiles within the skin. The increase in D-E junction humoral activity[24] is consistent with the reported increased in Th2-like cytokines such as IL-4 and IL-6 that promote and perpetuate B-cell hyperactivity and autoantibody formation while suppressing the production of Th1 cytokines in SLE.[45] By enhancing cell-mediated[17,18] and decreasing humoral-mediated[44] immunity, UV-A1 irradiation is well positioned to be therapeutic. The peroxidation of membrane lipids by these long wavelengths alters cell membranes sufficiently to alter cykotine release.[43] To date, although cytokine studies support the potential for UV-B[46] and possibly high-dose UV-A1[17] radiation to exacerbate this Th2-like profile, none describe the effects of low-dose UV-A1 irradiation on cytokines.

A recently described unique *in vitro* action of UV-A1 photons that has remedial potential is the induction of immediate apoptosis.[19] A form of programmed cell death directed at eliminating cells that are no longer necessary for or that may interfere with normal human development, apoptosis appears to be defective, blocked, or inhibited in SLE.[47] Although all UV wavelengths induce delayed transcriptional apoptosis, only those of UV-A1, through the generation of reactive oxygen species, bring about immediate non-transcriptional apoptosis.[20] Acting in a supplemental or preemptive mode in SLE, this relatively clean and noninflammatory type of programmed cell death would seem preferable to the alternatives: liquefaction degeneration and necrosis[24,48] with spillover of phlogistic cellular constituents into the circulation, or non-death leading to persistence and proliferation of activated autoimmune lymphocytes.[48]

The reciprocal propensities of UV-B and UV-A1 radiation may be reflected also in the recently described proclivity of UV-B but not UV-A photons to promote the translocation of soluble non-histone nuclear antigens, such as 52 and 60 kilodalton SSA, calreticulum, SSB, Sm, and RNP to the surface of cells.[22,23,49] These translocated intracellular antigens may then react with their respective antibodies in SLE patients, engendering ADCC,[40] with resulting disruption of the cell and escape of the antigens and various inflammatory constituents into the circulation; alternatively, the bound antibodies may undergo pinocytosis,[50] possibly accounting for the intraepidermal deposits of IgG found in SCLE.[38] The resolution of SCLE,[12,13] a disorder linked to the translocation phenomenon,[50] and the decrease in SSA antibody following UV-A1 exposures suggest that these wavelengths have an inhibitory effect on translocation. The failure of UV-A radiation, a combination of UV-A2 and UV-A1, to elicit translocation further implicates UV-A1 as inhibitory, since UV-A2 as a functional extension of UV-B, would be expected to effect some degree of translocation.

Viruses, SLE, and UV-A1 radiation

There are other agents that exacerbate SLE and promote translocation. Among these are estrdiol[51,52] and stress proteins.[53,54] But the more provocative are viruses. These trigger translocation[55,56] and have been linked etiologically to SLE; tubuloreticular structures have been identified in a variety of tissues,[57,58] including skin cells in which viruses' presence was enhanced by UV-B irradiation.[57] Anti-lymphocyte[59] and anti-dsDNA antibodies,[60] both close to pathognomonic in SLE, have been reported in laboratory workers handling SLE sera; evidence for a horizontally-transmittable agent also has been found in dogs with lupus.[61] The capacity for viruses to trigger translocation[55,56] seems a reasonable means by which they could escape capture through apoptosis: antigen translocation prior to apoptosis would predispose to destruction of the infected cell and release of the virus into the skin and circulation. Viruses are even known to directly inhibit apoptosis.[62] The fostering of immediate apoptosis by UV-A1 irradiation in this setting would act to preempt viral-induced translocation-triggered necrosis, offering a means by which UV-A1 photons might ameliorate disease activity in SLE and, even more, SCLE.

Inhibition of UV-B toxicity by UV-A1 photons

To be considered also is the possibility that UV-A1, in so many ways antagonistic to UV-B, engenders its benefits through exactly that means. All human subjects are consistently exposed to low levels of UV-B irradiation, whether from indirect sun exposure or artificial lighting. These low-dose exposures are sufficient to bring about UV-B-dependent activation of epidermal immunologic mediators *in vitro*,[63] and have been demonstrated to exacerbate SLE in human subjects.[64] Because UV-A1 exposures, directly inhibit UV-B photon action or correct impaired tolerance to UV-B photons[65] (akin to the treatment of polymorphous light eruption with psoralens and UV-A),[66] it may in this way modify disease in UV-B-sensitive SLE patients. In short, UV-A1 irradiation may well bring about at least a portion of its benefits by undermining the actions of UV-B.

A placebo controlled study

To confirm the effectiveness and safety of daily low-dose UV-A1 irradiation as a therapeutic agent in SLE, we enrolled 26 women with SLE in an 18 week two-phase study.[67] During an initial six week prospective, double-blind, placebo-controlled phase, patients were divided into two groups. Group A patients were exposed within a sunbed to 60 kJ/m² of

UV-A1 irradiation five days a week for three weeks and Group B patients for an equal amount of time to visible (placebo) light of greater than > 430 nm. Each group was then crossed over for exposure to the other source for three weeks. During a 12 week second phase, patients and physicians were unblinded and patients irradiated with progressively decreasing levels of only UV-A1.

The systemic lupus activity measure (SLAM)[68] score improved significantly in Group A patients after three weeks of five day a week UV-A1 irradiation ($P < 0.05$), regressing all the way to baseline during the three weeks of placebo irradiation. Improvement recurred and progressed during the six weeks of three day a week UV-A1 irradiation ($P < 0.05$). Group B patients responded negligibly to the three weeks of visible light, sharply to UV-A1, and, as with those in group A, maximally to the six weeks of three day a week UV-A1 ($P < 0.01$). With twice- and then once-weekly UV-A1 irradiation, SLAM scores began to worsen. All patients decreased their drug use. Anti-double-stranded DNA antibodies (anti-dsDNA) decreased significantly ($P < 0.05$) and anti-nuclear antibodies non-significantly. Side effects were negligible. Visible light had no significant effect. In short, then, low-dose UV-A1 irradiation effectively, comfortably, and without apparent toxicity, diminished signs and symptoms of disease activity in SLE.

UV-A1 action in fibromyalgia and rheumatoid arthritis

In this and the earlier studies, the most gratifying result of treatment for the majority of the patients was reversal of the profound fatigue that characterizes SLE. Since fibromyalgia is common in SLE and associated with high levels of fatigue, we tested a group of six patients with primary fibromyalgia but without SLE. We found them essentially unresponsive to the UV-A1 radiation therapy (unpublished data). Moreover, the patients with fatigue due to SLE had joint pain and tenderness rather than tenderness at the sites typical for fibromyalgia.[69] Anecdotally, one of our SLE study patients who suffered from both disorders insisted that she could tell the difference and reported that the UV-A1 therapy helped only the fatigue due to her SLE.

We also tested the action of UV-A1 on a group of six patients with rheumatoid arthritis and found no improvement (unpublished data). This disorder, like chronic cutaneous lupus, is cell-mediated, lending support to our impression that UV-A1 photons are not beneficial in cell-mediated disorders. On the other hand, three week exposures to black lamps emitting generous amounts of UV-B radiation that suppresses CMI had brought significant relief to a group of 26 rheumatoid arthritis patients.[70]

Effectiveness of long term UV-A1 radiation therapy

We followed the progress of six SLE patients for an average of 3.4 (range 2.4-4.5) years, using 2-3 irradiations of 6-15J/m² each (15-30 minutes or approximately 1/8-1/4 of the minimal erythema dose) per week.[71] These six had experienced significant decreases in signs and symptoms of disease activity during the first 12 weeks of earlier studies while receiving 3-5 treatments of low-dose UV-A1 irradiation, and had asked to continue on to long-term therapy. We assessed progress every three months with the SLAM. Despite the smaller number of weekly treatments, the significant gains achieved during the initial 12 weeks of the earlier studies persisted or increased. Additionally, we observed, as we had in the short-term studies, that patients experienced disease flares during occasional unavoidable 1-2 week omissions of UV-A1 therapy and that tanning was modest to negligible. We concluded that UV-A1-induced remissions in SLE persist over the longterm, with 1-2 weekly exposures sufficing and remissions remaining UV-A1 therapy-dependent. However, patients must be reminded that despite their feeling better, the disease requires the same close monitoring as was required before they began therapy.

The progressive albeit marginal improvement in the SLAM score in this long-term study brought to the fore the possibility that continued therapy would eventuate in permanent disease resolution. The course of one patient, DS longest in therapy, fostered this hope. Early on, the severe fatigue and photosensitivity that had kept her virtually house-bound abated as her anti-SSA antibody became negative. She began for the first time in years to work an eight hour day, and now, four years later, continues to do so, having discontinued her treatments four months earlier.

The risks: 1. melanoma

A potential danger of any long-term UV irradiation exposure is the development of skin tumors. Although relatively free of the risk of triggering basal or squamous cell tumors, UV-A wavelengths have been implicated in the generation of melanoma. A high proportion of the Xiphophorus genus of fish developed melanoma after a single exposure to UV and visible radiation with wavelengths within the UVA and visible spectrum contributing over 90% of the energy required.[72] In humans, epidemiologic data show that countries with the highest incidence of melanoma have the highest sunscreen use,[73] suggesting that the longer wavelengths of UV light — those not blocked by most sunscreens — are responsible. Finally, tanning parlors with lamps emitting high levels of UV-A and moderate levels of UV-B radiation have been linked to the genesis of melanoma.[74]

Conversely, sequence analysis of the CDKN2 tumor suppressor gene provides evidence against a significant role for UV-A in melanoma induction.[75] Also, recent studies attribute melanoma production in humans and animals to the shorter UV wavelengths and to intermittent sunlight exposures.[76] Moreover, the 'UV-A' radiation used for earlier studies associating irradiation with melanoma contained UV-A2 or UV-B. To date, there are no reports of UV-A1-induced tumor induction in humans, even after the high doses used in the treatment of atopic dermatitis,[17] much less with the low doses required in our studies.

Nevertheless, one of our patients, fair-skinned, red-haired, and non-sun-exposed, developed several enlarging lentigos after several years of twice-weekly UV-A1 exposures sufficient to produce a modest tan. Although three dermatologists assured us that the dysplastic changes seen on biopsy of two of these lesions were consistent with the picture of a 38 year old woman suddenly exposed to UV light (she was no longer sun-sensitive), we opted to discontinue her therapy rather than face the prospect of repeated biopsies. All our patients see dermatologists regularly, and there has been no other need for biopsy.

The risks: 2. photosensitivity

There are now reports of both UV-A and UV-A1 toxicity in SLE patients, with exposures inducing early, persistent erythema and sometimes rashes. However, the wavelengths used in these studies[77,78,79,80] differed from our own. One group of investigators irradiated patients with levels of UV-A an order of magnitude higher than our UV-A1 levels and inclusive of UV-A2 (320-340 nm),[77] the band now considered to be functionally an extension of UV-B.[9] A recently published case report on phototoxicity due to UV-A emissions from a photocopier machine[78] can be explained similarly. In a third study,[79] investigators elicited rashes only by employing monochromatic wavelengths approximately two orders of magnitude greater in intensity than any individual wavelength within our polychromatic UV-A1 spectrum. In a fourth study, UV-A wavelengths were found to be without toxicity.[80] We had only one patient drop out of our controlled study and that because of a photosensitive rash attributed to diltiazam, a photo-sensitizing drug that could not be replaced because of the patient's many drug allergies.

CONCLUSION

As opposed to virtually all other therapeutic modalities in SLE, UV-A1 photons delivered dermally at low levels, effectively, comfortably, progressively, and without apparent side effects, relieved constitutional and other signs and symptoms of disease activity, reduced the need for medication, and attenuated autoimmune antibody levels. We propose that these deeply penetrating photons implement their benefits primarily by quelling simmering inflammation within the skin, a massive organ that can contribute considerable phlogistic overflow in SLE. Possibly, too, although not addressed in these pages, the deeply penetrating UV-A1 photons[5] effect a more direct systemic 'reach' by acting on peripheral mononuclear cells circulating and percolating throughout the epidermis. The action of this therapy is not mediated through the eyes, since the opaque glasses worn by the patients preclude the entrainment of the optic-pineal-hypothalamic pathways that presumably occurs in a bright-light therapy for seasonal affective disorders.[81] The effectiveness of UV-A1 radiation therapy is provocative, offering not only a new mode of therapy but a new perspective on the complex role of ultraviolet light in this disorder.

REFERENCES

1. Cripps DJ, Rankin J. Action Spectra of lupus erythematosus and experimental immunofluorescence. *Arch Dermatol* 1973; **107**; 563-457.

2. Kochevar IE. Action spectrum and mechanisms of UV radiation induced injury in lupus erythematosus. *J Invest Dermatol* 1985; **85**; 14S-143S.

3.   Sutherland JC, Griffen KP. Absorption spectrum of DNA for wavelengths longer than 320 nm. *Radiat Res* 1981; **86**; 399-409.

4.   Bruls WAG *et al.* Transmission of human epidermis and stratum corneum as a function of thickness in the ultraviolet and visible wavelengths. *Photochem Photobiol* 1984; **40**; 485-494.

5.   Harm H. Damage and repair in mammalian cells after exposure to non-ionizing radiations III. Ultraviolet and visible light irradiation of cells of placental mammals, including humans, and determination of photorepairable damages in vitro. *Mutat Res* 1980; **69**; 167-176.

6.   Morison WL. The effects of UVA radiation on immune function (abstract). *Photochem Photobiol* 1985; **41 (suppl)**; 6S.

7.   McGrath H Jr, Bak E, Michalski JP. Ultraviolet A light prolongs survival and improves immune function in (New Zealand Black x New Zealand White)F_1 hybrid mice. *Arthritis Rheum* 1987; **30**; 557-561.

8.   Dixon FJ. Murine lupus: a model for human autoimmunity. *Arthritis Rheum* 1985; **28**; 1081-1088.

9.   Kochevar IE. Acute effects of ultraviolet radiation on skin. In: Holick MF, Kligman Am (eds). *Biologic Effects of Light*, Walter DeGruyter: New York, 1992, pp 1-10.

10.   McGrath H Jr., Bell MR, Haynes MR, Martinez, Osuna P. Ultraviolet_A irradiation therapy for patients with systemic lupus erythematosus: a pilot study. *Curr Ther Res* 1994; **55**; 373-381.

11.   Rivers JK. UVA sunbeds: tanning, photoprotection, acute and adverse effects and immunological changes. *Br J Dermatol* 1989; **120**; 767-777.

12.   McGrath H Jr. Ultraviolet-A1 irradiation decreases clinical disease activity and autoantibodies in patients with systemic lupus erythematosus. *Clin Exp Rheum* 1994; **12**; 129-135.

13.   Sonnichsen NH, Meffert V, Kunzelmann V, Audring H, UV-A1 therapy of subacute cutaneous lupus erythematosus. *Hautarzt* 1993; **44**; 723-725.

14. Lee LA. Neonatal lupus erythematosus. *J Invest Dermatol* 1993; **100**; 9S-13S.

15. Scopelitis E, Perez M, Biundo J. Anti-SSA antibody: a connective tissue disease marker. *J Rheumatol* 1985; **12**; 1105-1108.

16. Sutherland BM, Bennett PV. Human white blood cells contain cyclobutyl pyrimidine dimer photolyase. *Proc Natl Acad Sci USA* 1995; **92**; 9732-9736.

17. Krutmann J *et al.* High-dose UVA1 therapy in the treatment of patients with atopic dermatis. *J Am Acad Dermatol* 1992; **26**; 225-230.

18. Hager ED *et al.* Verbesserung Zellvermittelter immunitat bei tumopatienten durch hochdosierte phototerapie mit langwelligam ultraviolet-A (UV-A). *Dtsche z Onkol* 1989; **21**; 43-49.

19. Brainard GC *et al.* Ultraviolet regulation of neuroendocrine and circadian physiology in rodents and the visual evoked response in children. In: Urbach F (ed). *Physiological Effects of UV-A Radiation.* Valdenmar Publishing Co.; Overland Park, Kansas, 1992, pp 261-272.

20. Godar DE, Lucas AD. Spectral dependence of UV-induced immediate and delayed apoptosis: the role of membrane and DNA damage. *Photochem Photobiol* 1995; **62**; 108-113.

21. Grewe MK, Gyufko K, Krutmann J. Interleukin-10 production by cultured human keratinocytes: regulation by ultraviolet B and A1 radiation. *J Invest Dermatol* 1995; **104**; 3-6.

22. Golan TD, Elkon KB, Gharavi AE, Krueger JG. Enhanced membrane binding of autoantibodies to cultured keratinocytes of systemic lupus erythematosus patients after ultraviolet A/B irradiation. *J Clin Invest* 1992; **90**; 1067-1072.

23. Jones SK. Ultraviolet light (UVL) induction of cell-surface extractable nuclear antigen expression on human keratinocytes *in vitro*; a possible mechanism for the UVL induction of cutaneous lupus lesions *in vivo*. *Br J Dermatol* 1992; **126**; 554-560.

24. Tuffanelli DL, Kay D, Fukuyama K. Dermal-epidermal junction in lupus erythematosus. *Arch Dermatol* 1969; **99**; 652-662.

25. Setlow RB. Wavelengths in sunlight effective in producing skin cancer. A theoretical analysis. *Proc Natl Acad Sci USA* 1974; **71**; 3363-3366.

26. Tan EM, Schur PH, Carr RI, Kunkel HG. Deoxyribonucleic acid (DNA) and antibodies to DNA in the serum of patients with systemic lupus erythematosus. *J Clin Invest* 1966; **45**; 1732-1740.

27. Sutherland BM. Mutagenic lesions in carcinogenesis: induction and repair of pyrimidine dimers. *Photochemistry and Photobiology* 1996; **63**; 37S.

28. Tan EM. In: Miescher RA (ed). *Immunopathology: Sixth International Symposium.* Schwabe: Basil, 1971, pp 36-38.

29. Golan D, Borel Y. Spontaneous increase of DNA turnover in murine systemic lupus erythematosus. *E J Immunol* 1983; **3**; 430-433.

30. Davis P, Russel AS, Percy JS. Antibodies to UV light denatured DNA in systemic lupus erythematosus. *J Rheumatol* 1976; **3**; 375-379.

31. Horowitz DA. Impaired delayed type hypersensitivity in systemic lupus erythematosus. *Arthritis Rheum* 1972; **15**; 353-359.

32. Kripke ML, Applegate LW. Alterations in the immune response by ultraviolet radiation. In: Goldsmith LA (ed). *Physiology, Biochemistry and Molecular Biology of the Skin*, 2nd end. Oxford University Press: New York, 1991, pp 1222-1239.

33. Baadsgaard O, Wulf HC, Wantzin GL, Cooper KD. UVB and UVC, but not UVA, potently induce the appearance of T6 — DR + antigen-presenting cells in human epidermis. *J Invest Dermatol* 1987; **89**; 113-118.

34. DeFabo EC, Reilly DC, Noonan FP. Mechanism of UVA effects on immune function: preliminary studies: In: Urbach FA (ed). *Biologic Responses to UVA Radiation.* Valdenmar: Kansas City, 1991, pp 227-237.

35. Kim TY, Kripke ML, Ullrich SE. Immunosuppression by factors released from UV-irradiated epidermal cells: selective effects on the generation of contact and delayed hypersensitivities after exposures to UVA or UVB radiation. *J Invest Dermatol* 1990; **94**; 26-32.

36. Synkowski DR, Provost TT. Characterization of the inflammation in lupus erythematosus lesions using monoclonal antibodies. *J Rheumatol* 1983; **10**; 920-924.

37. Sonetheimer RD *et al.* Serologic and HLA associations of subacute cutaneous lupus erythematosus, a clinical subset of lupus erythematosus *Ann Intern Med* 1982; **97**; 664-671.

38. Nieboer C, Tak-Diamand Z, VanLeeuwen-Wallau AG. Dust-like particles: a specific direct immunofluorescence pattern in subacute cutaneous lupus erythematosus. *Br J Dermatol* 1988; **118**; 725-734.

39. Mascaro Jr. JM *et al.* Membrane attack complex deposits in cutaneous lesions of dermatomyositis. *Arch Dermatol* 1995; **131**; 1386-1392.

40. Norris DA *et al.* The role of RNP, Sm and SS-A/RO-Specific Antisera from patients with lupus erythematosus in inducing antibody-dependent cellular cytotoxicity (ADCC) of targets coated with nonhistone nuclear antigens. *Clin Immunol Immunopathol* 1984; **31**; 311-320.

41. Via CS *et al.* T cell-antigen-presenting cell interactions in human systemic lupus erythematosus: evidence for heterogeneous expression of multiple defects. *J Immunol* 1993; **151**; 3914-3922.

42. Simon JC, Cruz PD, Bergstresser PR, TIgelaar RE. Low dose UVB-irradiated Langerhans cells preferentially active CD4 cells of the Th1 subset. *J Immunol* 1990; **145**; 2087-2091.

43. Handwerger BS, Rus V, da Silva L, Via CS. The role of cytokines in the immunopathogenesis of lupus. *Springer Semin Immunopathol* 1994; **16**; 153-180.

44. Godar DE, Beer JZ. UVA-1 induced anuclear damage in mammalian cells. In: Urbach FA (ed). *Biologic Responses to Ultraviolet A Radiation*. Valdenmar: Kansas, 1991, pp 65-73.

45. Tyrrell RM. The Molecular and Cellular Pathology of Solar Ultraviolet Radiation. *Molec Aspects Med* 1994; **15**; 1-77.

46. Lugar TA, Schwartz T. Effects of UV light on cytokines and neuroendocrine hormones. In: Krutmann J, Elmets CA (eds). *Photoimmunology*. Blackwell Science Ltd: London, 1995, pp 55-76.

47. Carron DA, Tan EM. apoptosis in rheumatic disease. *Bull Rheum Dis* 1995; **44**; 1-3.

48. Searle J, Kerr JFR, Bishop CJ. Necrosis and apoptosis: distinct modes of cell death with fundamentally different significance. *Pathol Annu* 1982; **17 (pt 2)**; 229-259.

49. Kawashima T, Zappi, EG, Lieu TS, Sontheimer RD. Impact of Ultraviolet Radiation on the cellular expression of Ro/SS-A-autoantigenic polypeptides. *Dermatology* **189 (suppl. 1)**; 6-10.

50. Bajar KMD. Subacute cutaneous lupus erythematosus. *J Invest Dermatol* 1993; **100**; 2S-8S.

51. Lahita RG, Bradlow HL, Kunkel HG, Fishman J. Increased 16-alpha-hydroxylation of estradiol in systemic lupus erythematosus. *J Clin Endocrinol Metab* 1981; **53**; 174-178.

52. Furukawa *et al.* Estradiol enhances binding to cultured human keratinocytes of antibodies specific for SS-A/Ro and SS-B/La. *J Immunol* 1988; **141**; 1480-1488.

53. Winfield JB. Stress proteins, arthritis, and autoimmunity. *Arthritis Rheum* 1989; **32**; 1497-1504.

54. Kaufmann SHE. Heat shock proteins and the immune response. *Immunol Today* 1990; **11**; 129-136.

55. Baboonian C *et al.* Virus infection induces redistribution and membrane localization of the nuclear antigen La (SS-B): a possible mechanism for autoimmunity. *Clin Exp Immunol* 1989; **78**; 454-459.

56. Bachmann M *et al.* Translocation of the nuclear autoantigen La to the cell surface of herpes simplex virus type 1 infected cells. *Autoimmunity* 1992; **12**; 37-45.

57. Berk SH, Blank H. Ultraviolet light and cytoplasmic tubules in lupus erythematosus. *Arch Dermatol* 1974; **109**; 364-366.

58. Schumacher HR Jr, Howe HS. Synovial fluid cells in systemic lupus erythematosus: light and electron microscopic studies. *Lupus* 1995; **4**; 353-364.

59. DeHoratias RJ. Lymphocytoxic antibodies. *Prog Clin Immunol* 1980; **4**; 151-154.

60. Zarmbinski MA, Messner RP, Mandal JS. Anti-dsDNA antibodies in laboratory workers handling blood from patients with systemic lupus erythematosus. *J Rheumatol* 1992; **19**; 1380-1384.

61. Lewis RM *et al.* Canine systemic lupus erythematosus: Transmission of serologic abnormalities by cell-free filtrates. *J Clin Invest* 1973; **52**; 1893-1907.

62. Heinkelein M, Pilz S, Jassoy C. Inhibition of CD 95 (Fas/Apol)-mediated apoptosis by vaccinia virus WR. *Clin Exp Immunol* 1996; **103**; 8-14.

63. Rihner M, McGrath, Jr. H. Fluorescent light photosensitivity in patients with systemic lupus erythematosus. *Arthritis Rhem* 1992; **35**; 949-952.

64. McGrath H Jr, Bak E, Zimny ML, Michalski JB. Fluorescent light decreases autoimmunity and improves immunity in B/W mice. *J Clin Lab Immunol* 1990; **32**; 113-116.

65. Baadsgaard O. *In vivo* ultraviolet irradiation of human skin results in profound perturbation of the immune system: relevance to ultraviolet-induced skin cancer. *Arch Dermatol* 1991; **127**; 99-109.

66. Murphy GM *et al.* Prophylactic PUVA and UVB therapy in polymorphic light eruption: a controlled trial. *Br J Dermatol* 1987; **116**; 531-538.

67. McGrath H Jr, Martinez-Osuna P, Akdamar LF. Ultraviolet-A1 (340 nm) irradiation therapy in systemic lupus erythematosus. *Lupus* 1996; **5**; 269-274.

68. Liang MH, Socher SA, Larson MG, Schur PH. Reliability and validity of six systems for the clinical assessment of disease activity in SLE. *Arthritis Rheum* 1989; **32**; 1107-1118.

69. Wolfe F. Fibromyagia: a clinical syndrome. *Rheum Dis Clin NA* 1989; **15**; 1-17.

70. McGrath H Jr, Smith JL, Bak E, Michalski JP. Ultraviolet_A light in the treatment of rheumatoid arthritis. *Clin Exp Rheumatol* 1987; **5**; 323-328.

71. Molina JF, McGrath H Jr. Long-term UV-A1 irradiation in SLE. *Arthritis Rheum* 1995; **38**; S303.

72.   Setlow RB, Grist, Thompson K, Woodhead AD. Wavelengths effective in induction of malignant melanoma. *Proc Natl Acad Sci USA* 1992; **90**; 6666-6670.

73.   Garland CF, Garland FC, Gorham ED. Could sunscreens increase melanoma risk? *Am J Public Health* 1992; **82**; 614-615.

74.   Diffey BL, Farr PM. Tanning with UVB or UVA: an appraisal of risks. *J Photochem Photobiol B* 1991; **8**; 219-223.

75.   Pollock PM *et al.* Evidence for UV induction of CDKN2 mutations in melanoma cell lines. *Oncogene* 1995; **11**; 663-668.

76.   Armstrong BK, Kricker A. How much melanoma is caused by sun exposure? *Melanoma Res* 1992; **3**; 395-401.

77.   Lehmann P *et al.* Experimental reproduction of skin lesions in lupus erythematosus by UVA and UVB radiation. *J Am Acad Dermatol* 1989; **22**; 181-187.

78.   Klein LR, Elmets CA, Callen JP. Photoexacerbation of cutaneous lupus erythematosus due to ultraviolet A emissions from a photocopier. *Arthritis Rheum* 1995; **38**; 1152-1156.

79.   Nived O, Johansen PB, Sturfelt G. Standardized ultraviolet-A exposure provokes skin reaction in systemic lupus erythematosus. *Lupus* 1993; **2**; 247-250.

80.   Wolska H, Blaszczyk M, Jablonska S. Phototests in patients with various forms of lupus erythematosus. *Int J Dermatol* 1989; 98-102.

81.   Terman M, Terman JS. Light therapy for winter depression. In: Holick MF, Klugman AM (eds). *Biologic Effects of Light.* Walter de Gruyter & Co: New York, 1992, pp 171-187.

REVERSAL OF BRAIN DYSFUNCTION WITH UV-A1 IRRADIATION IN A PATIENT WITH SYSTEMIC LUPUS

Y Menon, K McCarthy and H McGrath Jr

Louisiana State University Medical School
New Orleans, Louisiana, USA

Source: Lupus 2003; 12, 479-482

Low-dose ultraviolet A-1 (UV-A1; 340-400 nm) bodily irradiation significantly reduces clinical manifestations of systemic lupus erythematosus (SLE). As neuropsychiatric-like symptoms respond prominently, a single patient was selected to undergo positron emission tomography (PET) before and after therapy to determine the effects of the therapy on the brain. The functional changes in ^{18}F-deoxyglucose uptake as determined by PET imaging in this SLE patient indicated that improvement in brain function paralleled the reversal of cognitive deficits noted after the administration 160 kJ of bodily UV-A1 irradiation administered three times a week. Also of interest is that the UV-A1 irradiation, for the first time, ameliorated discoid lupus rashes, presumably due to a systemic action, as the lesions were for the first time covered during therapy.

INTRODUCTION

Ultraviolet (UV) light sensitivity is characteristic of patients with systemic lupus erythematosus (SLE). Of the ultraviolet wavelengths, ultraviolet B (UVB 280-320 nm) wavelengths are the most toxic, UV-A2 (320-340 nm) wavelengths somewhat less so. Paradoxically, UV-A1 wavelengths, differing markedly in their properties from the shorter wavelengths, have proved to have a beneficial action in SLE. Low-dose bodily UV-A1 irradiation relieved arthritis, rashes and photosensitivity, and an array of neuropsychiatric-like symptoms in patients with SLE.[1,2,3,4] The favorable response of the neuropsychiatric-like symptoms such as migraine, headache, decreased concentration, disordered affect and depression[5] suggested an indirect action on the brain. To test for this, a single patient was selected for functional brain scanning with positron emission tomography (PET) before and after 24 weeks of UV-A1 irradiation therapy. An updated SLE measures (SLAM-2), a series of visual analog scales (VAS), and standard autoimmune laboratory tests together gauged concomitant clinical changes. The hypothesis that UV-A1 irradiation-induced improvement in the neuropsychiatric-like manifestations of SLE would correspond to improvement in brain metabolism as depicted by PET imaging proved valid in this patient.

CASE REPORT

A 37-year old Hispanic woman was diagnosed in 1995 with SLE after having presented with arthralgias, photosensitivity, pleurisy, depression, migraine headaches, and the presence of antinuclear and SSA antibodies. She was initially diagnosed as well with irritable bowel syndrome and fibromyalgia. Treatment with hydroxychloroquine, prednisone and antidepressants brought some relief. Before entering the study she complained of increasing memory loss, diminished concentration, depression, migraine headaches, fatigue and joint pain, all of which interfered with her daily activities, especially with her job as a paralegal. On physical examination she had mild tenderness over her metacarpophalangeal joints bilaterally, four to five tender points, and active discoid lesions within her left auditory canal, on her left ear lobe, and as a brownish-black 6 cm-diameter discoid patch, on her right tibia. Neuropsychiatric evaluation revealed a loss of short-term memory, mild cognitive impairment, depression and headache. Her antinuclear antibody titer was 1:320, complement levels normal, erythrocyte sedimentation rate 14 mm/h, and a complete blood count within normal limits.

Bodily UV-A1 irradiation, 160 kJ/m², approximately one-sixth of a minimal erythematous dose, was administered over 30 min three times a week for 24 weeks (except for weeks 12-14 following a back injury). The irradiator was a bench-and-canopy type fan-cooled sun bed fitted with a combination of lamps and filters that transmitted ultraviolet radiation solely in the UV-A1 range as previously described.[2] During the first 2-3 weeks of therapy the patient experienced marked improvement in her fatigue, joint pain, discoid rashes and in her memory, diminished concentration, and depression. She returned to work.

Prior to and 24 weeks after the initiation of therapy, she underwent whole-body PET scanning using 16.7mCi of [18]F 2 fluoro-2-deoxy-glucose. The PET scans were obtained using standardized cortical and subcortical elliptical regions of interest (ROIs) assigned to three adjacent transaxial slices of the following regions: frontal, parietal, occipitofrontal, temporolateral, temporomedial, parieto-occipital, thalamus, putamen, caudate nucleus, cerebellar (mean of lateral and dorsal cerebellum), brain stem and global at the level of the thalamus and basal ganglia. Shape and size were fitted to actual head form by computer simulation. The position of ROIs was adjusted to the corresponding anatomical localization. In each ROI, the average uptake per pixel per time was determined. ROI analysis was performed using a SUN sparc station and SUNVIEW software. To allow inter-individual comparisons, regional cerebral metabolism was normalized by global glucose metabolism (glucose metabolic index, GMI; GMI = ROI uptake) determined from the global brain ROI at the level of thalamus and basal ganglia.

The PET scan prior to therapy in reconstructed images of the brain revealed some subtle but apparently focal abnormalities involving the left posterior parietal cortex near the interhemispheric fissure. There was also an area of slightly diminished uptake in the right temporal lobe anteriorly. There were two small areas in the same location anteriorly in the left temporal lobe. In addition, there was noted to be somewhat diminished global uptake within the cerebellum compared with the remainder of the cortical gray matter. The results were significant for asymmetric and focally abnormal disparities in regional glucose metabolism in the left posterior parietal cortex near the interhemispheric fissure, cerebellum, and anteriorly in the right temporal lobe.

Following the 24 weeks of UV-A1 irradiation therapy a repeat PET scan showed a homogeneous pattern of uptake with complete clearing of the earlier described abnormalities. The SLAM improved from a score of 12 to 2. The VAS for fatigue improved from a score of 8 down to 2, diminished concentration from 8 to 2, depression from 8 to 5, joint pain from 6 to 3, discoid rash from 8 to 3, and headache remained unchanged at 4. This clinical improvement was experienced at 2-3 weeks and persisted beyond the date of the second PET. Photosensitivity decreased at 8-9 months.

DISCUSSION

This 34-year-old woman, after 2-3 weeks of 240 kJ/m² doses of UV-A1 irradiation administered three times a week, experienced rapid dimunition of discoid lupus lesions on her leg and ear and equally rapid diminishment of arthralgias, but most gratifyingly from the patient's viewpoint, marked attenuation of fatigue and of the neuropsychiatric-like symptoms of depression, memory loss and diminished concentration. These changes were persistent throughout 24 weeks of therapy. Although relief of these neuropsychiatric-like symptoms in SLE are experienced commonly during UV-A1 irradiation therapy, this was the first time an attempt was made to correlate them to the reversal of abnormalities in the brain as determined by PET. It is the first time that a chronic lupus (discoid) rash has responded to UV-A1 irradiation therapy, previously effective only for acute and sub-acute lupus rashes.[1,2,4] It was also the first time that a discoid rash was protected from direct UV-A1 exposure, suggesting that the response, like that of the joint pain, fatigue and neuropsychiatric-like symptoms, was systemically mediated.

Although gross pathology of the brain may be well visualized by conventional neuroimaging, recent studies suggest that any physiologic, metabolic or biochemical change may be better assessed by functional nuclide imaging. Whereas MRI is the technique of choice to define anatomy in neuropsychiatric SLE,[6] it is less likely to show abnormalities in patients with affective disorders, confusional states or headache.[7] The radionuclide technique of PET is best suited toward this end because of its unique ability to assess functional abnormalities of blood flow and metabolism. PET findings are often abnormal in patients with active neuropsychiatric SLE, demonstrating multiple focal defects in glucose uptake that may not be evident by CT or MRI.[8,9] In one study 100% of [18]FDG-PET scans from patients with active neuropsychiatric SLE showed abnormal results whereas only 15% of MRI scans showed abnormalities.[9] PET scans showed hypometabolism in at least one region of the brain in 100% of 26 SLE patients with severe or mild neuropsychiatric symptoms.[10] This sensitive technique permits an objective assessment of responses to the UV-A1 irradiation treatment beyond what is measured by improvement in central nervous system (CNS) signs and symptoms. In the present patient there were multiple abnormalities depicted on PET prior to therapy and none following therapy.

How might UV-A1 photon action on the skin reach an organ such as the brain, removed from this site? The skin is the largest organ in the body, intimately and extensively involved in SLE, and the immediate target of irradiation. Delivered through the skin, the UV-A1 photons have dermatologic and systemic actions, the latter in the present case possibly affecting the central nervous system. As blood traverses the dermis for only a few seconds approximately every 8 minutes,[11] the direct UV-A1 photon impact on blood elements has to be minimal. Moreover, there is no way for UV-A1 light to reach the brain directly as the eyes are covered during the therapy and there is no direct access through the skull because the UV-A1 photons penetrate only to the dermis.[12] Therefore, it is likely that the greater part or all of the resolution of the CNS-like manifestations of SLE is due to the photon-induced release, or interdiction of release, of mediators from the skin into the blood and to the brain.

The most likely site for this modulation is the dermal-epidermal junction, the most consistently immunoreactive and chronically simmering inflammatory site of involvement in SLE.[13] Unlike the shorter wavelengths, the deeply penetrating UV-A1 wavelengths readily reach this site,[12] where any dampening of disease activity through, for example, the promotion of apoptosis,[14] or the targeting of T cells,[15,16] could serve to reduce not only the dermal manifestations of disease but the constitutional, synovial and neuropsychiatric-like symptoms that result from changes in the efflux of phlogistic constituents from the dermal-epidermal junction into the circulation.

Of the environmental agents impacting on and processed by the skin, sunlight is unique. Having been intimately involved with human evolution for eons, the sun's photons orchestrate, through this massive organ, the release or inhibition of a myriad of mediators that diminish or promote expression of multiple systemic physiological actions. Although the advent of altering immunological and physiologic milieu of the body with biologic mediators has great potential, the harnessing of an environmental agent already accomplishing this for eons in a highly coordinated manner is an approach with equally great promise. In the present instance, exploitation of the complex but balanced properties of a defined portion of the UV spectrum has led to a focused, efficient and safe immunologic tool for patients with SLE.

In summary, UV-A1 photon therapy, reaching beyond its major target, the skin, brought symptomatic relief systematically, presumably due to a

modulatory action on immunomediator trafficking. Clinical ameliora-
tion of cognitive dysfunction correlated with metabolic changes in the
brain identified by ^{18}F-deoxyglucose imaging. Discoid rashes, covered
during the therapy and therefore apparently engaged also by a systemically mediated action, responded for the first time to UV-A1 photon
therapy.

ACKNOWLEDGEMENTS

This work was supported by the National Institutes of Health grant
RRO5096-06, the Tulane/LSU General Clinical Research Center,
Charity Hospital, New Orleans, LA, USA, and the Louisiana Lupus
Foundation, Baton Route, LA, USA. We also want to thank Sheila
Mason, our nurse co-ordinator.

REFERENCES

1. McGrath H. Ultraviolet-A1 irradiation decreases clinical disease
   activity and autoantibodies in patients with systemic lupus erythematosus. *Clin Exp Rheum* 1994; **12**: 129-135.

2. McGrath H Jr, Martinez-Osuna, P, Lee AK. Ultraviolet-A1 (340-
   400 nm) irradiation therapy in systemic lupus erythematosus.
   Lupus 1996; **5**: 269-274.

3. Molina JF, McGrath H Jr. Long-term UV-A1 irradiation in SLE.
   J Rheumatol 1997; **24**: 1072-1074.

4. Polderman MCA, Huizinga TWJ, Cessie SLE, Paval S. UVA-1
   cold light treatment of SLE: a double blind placebo controlled
   crossover trial. *Ann Rheum Dis* 2001; **60**: 112-115.

5. Singer J, Denburg, JA. ACR Ad Hoc Committee on
   Neuropsychiatric Lupus Nomenclature. The American College of
   Rheumatology and the Ad Hoc Neuropsychiatric Lupus
   Workshop Group. Diagnostic criteria for neuropsychiatric sys-
   temic lupus erythematosus: the results of a consensus meeting.
   Arthritis Rheum 1999; **42**: 599-608.

6. Stimmler MN, Coletti PM, Quismorio FP Jr. Magnetic reso-
   nance imaging of the brain in neuropsychiatric systemic lupus
   erythematosus. *Semin Arthritis Rheum* 1993; **22**: 335-349.

7.   West SG, Emlen Wm, Wener MH, Casein BL. Neuropsychiatric lupus erythematosus: a 10-year prospective study on the value of diagnostic tests. *Am J Med* 1995; **99**: 153-163.

8.   Carbotte RM, Denburg SD, Denburg JA, Nahmias C, Garnett E S. Fluctuating cognitive abnormalities and cerebral glucose metabolism in neuropsychiatric systemic lupus erythematosus. *J Neurol Neurosurg Rheum* 1998; **41**: 1141-1151.

9.   Otte A, Weiner SM, Peter HH, *et al.* Brain glucose utilization in systemic lupus erythematosus with neuropsychiatric symptoms: a controlled positron emission tomography study. *Eur J Nucl Med* 1997; **24**: 787-791.

10.   Weiner SM, Otte A, Schumacher M *et al.* Alterations of cerebral glucose metabolism indicate progress to severe morphological brain lesions in neuropsychiatric systemic lupus erythematosus. *Lupus* 2000; **59**: 377-385.

11.   Kraemer KH, Weinstein GD. Decreased thymidine incorporation in circulating leukocytes after treatment of psoriasis with psoralen and long wave ultraviolet light. *J Invest Dermatol* 1977; **69**: 211-214.

12.   Bruls WAG, Slaper H, Van Der Leun JS, Berrens I. Transmission of human epidermis and stratum corneum as a function of thickness in the ultraviolet and visible wavelengths. *Photochem Photobiol* 1984; **40**: 485-494.

13.   Tuffanelli DL, Kay D, Fukuyama K. Dermal-epidermal junction in lupus erythematosus. *Arch Dermatol* 1969; **99**: 652-662.

14.   Godar DE. UVA1 radiation triggers two different final apoptotic pathways. *J Invest Dermatol* 1999; **112**: 3-12.

15.   Krutman J, Elmets CA (eds). Ultraviolet-A1 radiation-induced immunomodulation: high dose UV-A1 therapy of atopic dermatitis. In *Photoimmunology*. Blackwell Science: Oxford, 1995, pp 246-256.

16.   Breuckmann F, von Kobyletgki G, Avermaete A, Krueter A, Altmeyer P. Efficacy of ultraviolet A1 phototherapy on the expression of bcl-1 in atopic dermatitis and cutaneous T-cell

lymphoma *in vivo*; a comparison study. *Photodermatol Photoimmunol Photomed* 2002; **18**: 217-222.

NORMALIZATION OF ANTICARDIOLIPIN ANTIBODY LEVELS USING UVA1 IRRADIATION

Poster Session Presentation by Hugh McGrath, Jr., M.D., at the 7th International Congress for SLE and Related Conditions, May 12, 2004, New York, New York

Ultraviolet-A1 (UV-A1; 340-400 nm) irradiation of SLE patients reduces arthritis, fatigue, rashes, photosensitivity, and, perhaps most notably, cognitive decline. A total of two patients suffering cognitive decline were selected for positron emission tomography (PET), before and after more than six months of low-dose UVA1 bodily irradiation. The first patient, previously reported in the literature, had reversal of cognitive dysfunction and total resolution of the metabolic dysfunction that had been depicted by diminished ^{18}F-deoxyglucose uptake on PET imaging.

The second patient, reported herein, was a 30 year-old woman with full criteria of SLE who had livedo reticularis, high levels of IgM anticardiolipin antibodies, and a five-year history of progressive memory and concentration loss. After 8 months of 11 J/cm² of UVA1 irradiation twice a week, this patient experienced cessation of the progression of her cognitive decline. Elevated IgM anticardiolipin antibodies decreased from 44 mpl U/mL (normal<10) to 37 mpl U/mL one month after initiation of therapy and to 8mpl U/mL after 8 months of therapy. PET scan depiction of an asymmetric reduction in ^{18}F-uptake in the right inferior parietal and temporal lobes remained stable.

As there is no previously known agent that lowers anticardiolipin antibody levels, the marked but gradual decrease of these antibodies to normal during UVA1 irradiation therapy in this SLE patient, associated with an apparent cessation of cognitive decline, is clearly hopeful and warrants further study.

UVA1 LIGHT TREATMENT OF SLE: A DOUBLE BLIND, PLACEBO CONTROLLED CROSSOVER TRIAL UVA-1 COLD LIGHT TREATMENT OF SLE: A DOUBLE BLIND, PLACEBO CONTROLLED CROSSOVER TRIAL

M.C.A. Polderman, Department of Dermatology, Leiden University Medical Centre, The Netherlands; T. W. J. Huizinga, Department of Rheumatology, Leiden University Medical Centre; S. Le Cessie, Department of Medical Statistics, Leiden University Medical Centre; S. Pavel, Department of Dermatology, Leiden University Medical Centre, The Netherlands.

Original, unedited source:
Annals of the Rheumatic Diseases, 2001; 60:112-115 (February)

OBJECTIVE — The medical treatment of systemic lupus erythematosus (SLE) patients often requires strong drugs that have potentially serious side effects. Consequently, there is a need for new immunosuppressive treatments. Long wave ultraviolet A (UVA1) light therapy is an anti-inflammatory, immunomodulatory treatment with a possible systemic effect and few side effects. In this study, low dose UVA1 light therapy was tested to determine whether or not it can reduce disease activity in SLE patients.

METHOD — Eleven SLE patients were treated with UVA1 light and a placebo light treatment in a double blind, placebo controlled, crossover study. In two consecutive 12 week periods the patients were treated in the first three weeks with UVA1 and the placebo treatment, or vice versa. The primary variables were the SLE Disease Activity Index (SLEDAI) and SLE Activity Measure (SLAM).

RESULTS — The mean SLAM and SLEDAI showed a significant decrease of 30.4 percent (p=0.0005) and 37.9 percent (p=0.016) respectively after three weeks of UVA1, and a non-significant decline of 9.3 percent (p=0.43) and 12.2 percent (p=0.54) respectively after three weeks of placebo treatment. In this small trial the difference in reduction of the disease activity indices during UVA1 compared with during placebo treatment failed to reach the conventional border of significance (p=0.07). The total score of quality of life measure RAND-36 did not improve significantly, but the subscore for vitality did improve.

CONCLUSION — Low dose UVA1 light treatment was strongly suggestive of lowering SLE disease activity in this double blind placebo controlled study, and no side effects occurred.

NEW FINDING SHEDS LIGHT ON MECHANISM OF INFLAMMATION IN LUPUS, OTHER DISORDERS

Press Release: September 4, 2003

Source: Duke University Medical Center;
Durham Veterans Administration Hospital

Durham, NC — New insights into how the body eliminates dead cells could lead to new approaches for treating conditions including lupus and cancer, or for preventing infections following trauma. Researchers at Duke University Medical Center and the Durham Veterans Administration Hospital say the specialized cells that clear dead cells from the body have a much more complicated — and important — role than scientists previously understood.

Most human cells die through a process known as apoptosis, or "programmed cell death," and are rapidly removed from the body. In contrast, necrotic death occurs when cells die from injury or disease. Increased amounts of DNA from dead cells can be measured in the blood following a wide range of medical events including trauma, heart attacks, blood clots to the lung and chemotherapy treatment. Best known as the molecule of heredity, DNA may perform other activities when it is released from dead cells and appears in the blood.

Dead cells are cleared from the body by macrophages, scavenger cells of the immune system. When macrophages do not remove dead cells, the contents of the dead cells, including the DNA, can trigger a response from the immune system, which may eventually weaken the body and leave it susceptible to infection, a common complication following trauma. For people with lupus, the contents of the dead cells, especially DNA, may form immune complexes with antibodies that can cause inflammation that is not only painful but also damaging to organs such as the kidneys.

Scientists have long believed DNA from dead cells is present in the bloodstream only when macrophages become overwhelmed with more dead cells than they can remove. In other words, the contents of the dead cells "overflow" from the macrophages. David Pisetsky, M.D., professor of medicine and chief of the division of rheumatology and immunology at Duke University Medical Center, and colleagues recently discovered this may not be the case. The Duke team reports their findings, from studies funded by the Alliance for Lupus Research in the Sept. 15, 2003, issue of the journal Blood.

The Duke team was surprised while performing a series of experiments to determine whether administration of a large amount of apoptotic and necrotic cells would cause an increased amount of DNA to appear in the blood of mice. In their first experiment, the researchers found that injecting mice with a large quantity of dead cells indeed resulted in increased DNA in the mice's blood.

In the next experiment, they engineered mice lacking macrophages and injected the mice with a large quantity of dead cells. Because macrophages were not present to remove the dead cells, the team expected to find all of the dead cell DNA in the bloodstream. Instead, they found none.

"This result was totally unexpected, and caused us to step back and consider how the macrophages function to remove cell waste," Pisetsky said. Without macrophages, his team eventually theorized, dead cells cannot be broken down efficiently enough for DNA to appear in the bloodstream at a detectable level. Cells not processed by macrophages and removed from the body may accumulate and cause inflammation.

"What we hypothesize is that uptake by macrophages is not just part of the process, but is absolutely crucial to the appearance of DNA from dead cells in the blood," Pisetsky said. "The macrophages can't be bypassed by the dead cells, even if there is more cell DNA than they can process."

According to the researchers, this would mean that DNA from dead cells appears in the blood only when macrophages "fill" to capacity and perhaps then die and release all of their contents, including the DNA from the engulfed cells.

"If we are indeed correct," said Pisetsky, "then macrophages play a much more crucial role than previously thought. This finding could potentially have implications for the treatment of lupus and other inflammatory conditions."

The researchers said macrophages might be reinforced to clear larger amounts of dead cells, thus reducing the amount of DNA and other cellular molecules that pass into the blood and cause inflammation. "This mechanism could apply not only to lupus, but also to conditions like cancer, where we often intentionally kill large numbers of cells with chemotherapy and other treatments," said Pisetsky.

Likewise, bolstering macrophages could help prevent the immune response following trauma, and thereby help the body maintain normal levels of immunity to prevent subsequent infection.

The findings also may lend new insight to the function of current lupus treatment with corticosteroids, the researchers said. "Corticosteroids are one of the standard treatments for inflammation in lupus. We've always thought the steroids worked by reducing inflammation, but it may be that, in fact, they strengthen the macrophages and prevent the inflammatory response from beginning," said Pisetsky.

Joining Pisetsky in this research were Ning Jiang, M.D., of the division of rheumatology and immunology at Duke University Medical Center, and Charles Reich of the division of rheumatology and immunology at the Durham Veterans Administration Hospital.

UVA1, UVB AND UNSHIELDED FLUORESCENT LIGHT EFFECTS ON SYSTEMIC LUPUS ERYTHEMATOSUS MICE: IMMUNOLOGICAL AND PATHOLOGICAL EXAMINATIONS

D.E. Godar, FDA, Rockville, MD; A.D. Lucas, FDA, Rockville, MD; T.W. Claggett, Pathology Associates International, Frederick, MD; J.W. Lee, Mentor Technologies, Inc., Lanham, MD; J. Zhang, FDA, Beltsville, MD.

Original, unedited source: U.S. Food and Drug Administration (www.cfsan.fda.gov/~frf/forum97/97105.htm)

Pilot human studies using filtered tanning lamps have suggested that UVA1 radiation (340-400 nm) can alleviate the autoimmune symptoms of systemic lupus erythematosus (SLE) patients. In order to test for potential health risks and benefits, we irradiated a SLE mouse model with 1) UVA1 radiation from filtered tanning lamps, 2) UVB radiation, and 3) fluorescent light (visible + UVA and UVB). The results indicated that low doses of UVA1 radiation (TL/10R bulbs), unlike UVB radiation (TL/01R bulbs), beneficially alters the immune status (increased CD8[+] suppressor T cells ($p<0.05$) without affecting CD4[+] helper T cells), but does not exacerbate kidney damage.

Printed in the United Kingdom
by Lightning Source UK Ltd.
105880UKS00001B/163